With much respect
and warmth

love

To Ray Wm Jr.

The most satisfactory son
a father could have.
Dad

THE
PSYCHIATRIC
FORUM

Contributors

MANFRED BLEULER
FRANCIS J. BRACELAND
NORMAN Q. BRILL
EUGENE B. BRODY
JOHN M. CALDWELL
A. M. DERSHOWITZ
HAMILTON F. FORD
ROBERT S. GARBER
ROBERT W. GIBSON
HANS HOFF
GUSTAV HOFMANN
LEO KANNER
EDWARD H. KNIGHT
GABRIEL LANGFELDT
FRANK H. LUTON
WILLIAM MALAMUD
JUDD MARMOR
PETER A. MARTIN
HERBERT C. MODLIN
FRANCIS J. O'NEILL
HOWARD P. ROME
HAROLD M. VISOTSKY
RAYMOND W. WAGGONER
JULIUS ZELLERMAYER

The Psychiatric Forum

Edited by

GENE USDIN, M.D.

Clinical Professor of Psychiatry and Biobehavioral Sciences
Louisiana State University School of Medicine

BRUNNER/MAZEL *Publishers* • New York
BUTTERWORTHS • London

*All royalties from this volume are being contributed
to the* AMERICAN PSYCHIATRIC MUSEUM, INC.

Reprinted with Permission of PSYCHIATRY DIGEST, INC.

Published by
BRUNNER/MAZEL, INC.
64 University Place
New York, N. Y. 10003

Library of Congress Catalog Card No. 75-173093
SBN 87630-045-X

MANUFACTURED IN THE UNITED STATES OF AMERICA

Introduction

In this age of accelerated change—the age of Toffler's "Future Shock"—which often demands immediate responses, innovation and dramatic actions, many problems of human behavior press for interum solution and cannot wait for the luxury of longer-term, orderly resolution by scientific validation or documentation. So great is the rush of history and its ever-changing patina of problems that we must often consider even intuitive hunches—particularly in the behavioral field.

To meet the situation, *Psychiatry Digest* initiated the Psychiatric Forum, a feature in which outstanding authorities could speak out freely on a wide variety of timely topics of their own choice. Topics chosen could, but need not have to, bear the scrutiny of careful scientific study and could be free from such encumbrances as weighty references. Topics were to be current and controversial and to reflect the convictions of the writer gained from years of professional experience. An inducement for both writer and reader was that the articles be brief.

Experts should be guided by the course of human events and their own sensitivity when the urgings of necessity prohibit the luxury of time for meditating alternative measures. Many experts, however, hesitate to speak overtly for fear of professional censure.

The Forum's purpose was to provide the opportunity for the expression of pungent free-flowing fantasies, notions, crusades, innovative concepts, and professional self-criticism. The hope was that these opinions might prove valuable if ventured into with the assurance that the medium of expression solicited and endorsed their speculative and hopefully provocative nature. The opinions expressed and conclusions drawn by the contributors are their own and do not necessssarily reflect those of the editors or publishers of *Psychiatry Digest*.

Many professionals trained in the tradition of the typical scientific format, i.e., review of literature, hypothesis, data, conclusions—welcome the opportunity for free unfettered self-expression. Indeed, since we have encouraged free-associative techniques in our work with patients, is it too much a license to occasionally bare our own professional souls in print?

The contributors to this volume expounded ideas they deemed especially vital ranging through autobiographical accounts, theoretical concepts of specific illnesses, cultural problems, appropriate responsibility and delivery of services, effects of modern medical technocracy and psychoanalytic principles in the treatment of severe and minor illnesses of the young and the old.

The Forums fell naturally into four sections—administrative, clinical, nature of psychiatry, and social psychiatry. This book contains those Forums which were considered to be of longer interest and omits those which were extremely brief or dealt with topics now less significantly relevant.

The wish is that this anthology will stimulate—will suggest new dimensions to problem solving, new areas of research and new approaches to therapy. Hopefully, it will alert the reader to pressing current issues, encourage deeper introspection and focus attention on some of the more critical areas to which behavioral scientists may apply the unique talents of their particular discipline.

GENE USDIN, M.D.

Contents

vii

SECTION II: SOCIAL PSYCHIATRY

SECTION III: ADMINISTRATION AND SERVICES

SECTION IV: NATURE OF PSYCHIATRY

Section I
CLINICAL PSYCHIATRY

The Genesis and Nature of Schizophrenia

MANFRED BLEULER, M.D.

Director, Psychiatric Clinic, University of Zurich

The genesis and nature of schizophrenic psychoses are still obscure. In any discussion on the subject one is confronted with difficult, multifaceted, and hotly disputed problems. If I have to take a position in only a few pages, it cannot be done without simplifications which may sometimes stretch the limits of the permissible. Peremptory statements must be made on subjects which should be formulated with great caution and hedged by many "ifs" and "buts." I can only justify the presentation in print of the observations which follow after I have emphasized these reservations.

The term "schizophrenia" is so much abused nowadays that we must give a brief description of what we mean by this designation in our own outline. In the main, I follow the meaning of the term as it has been interpreted by Eugen Bleuler, a concept which has now found wide (but not general) acceptance in psychiatric thinking: Schizophrenia is a psychosis—a genuine mental illness; minor disturbances (e.g., neurasthenic disturbances) should not be designated as schizophrenia when they have never attained the degree of a psychosis. What is a psychosis and a mental illness? Just what it is only results from the experience of a mentally healthy person with himself and his healthy life companions. On the basis of this experience we understand and grasp the very essence of our fellow creatures in a quite definite frame of reference. We understand what he says and guess what he thinks; we can conjecture what he perceives and what he does not perceive; we can recognize the principal motives of his actions and can predict them in many situations; approximately, we can tell what he will and what he will not do; we can feel with him in many of his sensations and emotions. In some individuals this is no longer so. They still speak the same language, but we no longer understand them; they perceive impressions that we do not perceive and vice versa; their actions are incomprehensible; their moods, their emotional utterances of mourning or joy are strange to us. They have removed themselves from ordinary relationships, moved far away and have anchored themselves there; they are "out of joint," psychotic, mentally ill.

Schizophrenias are mental diseases but which mental diseases are schizophrenias? In the negative we can state the following: Mental diseases marked by primary disturbances of perception and memory, and by mere impoverishment and simplification of all psychic life, are not schizophrenias. (They are sequelae of brain diseases.) Nor are psychic disturbances, in which acute diminution of psychic life is of the essence (lethargy, subcoma conditions, coma), properly referred to as schizophrenia. Psychoses, which can be interpreted as exaggerations of a uniform mood are likewise not schizophrenias. Positively, we can say that schizophrenias are psychoses where the healthy psychic life is hidden behind the psychotic experience or proceeding side by side with it. Elementary disturbances concern disorderly thinking, feeling, and depersonalization. These are aspects of one and the same disturbance affecting the entire personality. Once the thought processes have become disorderly, one can no longer have uniform emotions, and once order and harmony between thinking and feeling have been lost, one can no longer perceive oneself as the uniform person one once was. All other symptoms seen in schizophrenic psychoses (e.g., hallucinations, delusions, secondary memory lapses, disturbed motor activity) are merely aspects of the same basic disturbance.

The terms "dementia praecox" (Kraepelin, 1899) and "schizophrenic psychoses" (Eugen Bleuler, 1911) were coined in a time when it was natural for people to search for uniform disease syndromes. There was a strong tendency to present pathology as a sum of "disease units." Each disturbance was supposed to be a unit in a disease, with its own etiology, own symptomatology, course, own therapy, and prophylaxis. In particular did such an endeavor suggest itself to the psychiatrist in view of the fact that it had been possible a few decades earlier to delineate diseases which seemed to approach the ideal of a disease unit: progressive paralysis, delirium tremens, alcohol hallucinosis. It was also at that time that Mendel's theory of heredity was taken over by psychiatry. It suggested the idea that a certain gene was responsible for a certain disease. Infectious diseases had been described according to definite pathogens earlier. But the attempt to uncover certain disease units and to classify them systematically is much older. It already guided the thinking of the classic French school of psychiatry at the beginning of the last century—of men like Pinel and Esquirol. It leaned on the comprehensive concept of a *systema naturae* of Linné and others. In the last resort these attempts stem from the spiritual need of man to classify the world, to oversee it and rule it, a requirement that is basic for the mental development of humanity. Of course, this desire has also led them into dead-end alleys; for instance when the ancients invented a system of psychoses where each psychosis corresponded to a characteristic demon.

Nothing was more natural—and more necessary—than that the hypothesis "one disease, one cause" was elevated to the guiding principle of schizophrenia research.

Hence, research proceeded accordingly. Workers searched for one cause for each disease, one gene, a definite intoxication, a definite "inborn error of metabolism," a definite psychic trauma during a specific phase of development. However, no such uniform cause was unearthed. Generations of research workers seemed to have wasted their time and people spoke of a "scandal of psychiatry."

Now, however, it is becoming more and more evident that multiple damages may cooperate in the development of diseases. We must not lose heart if we do not discover a single decisive cause. This search for a single, or at most a few decisive, specific causes of the disease, has—in the research of schizophrenia—hampered the study of its pathogenesis for a long time, because it is affected by a multiplicity of influences.

Further obstacles also stood in the way of clarifying the nature of schizophrenia. Until recently all hypotheses were based on a few isolated findings. Only very few who erected these hypotheses took all important aspects of schizophrenic psychosis into account.

I will briefly summarize the most important conditioning factors which one ought to consider foremost when one builds up a hypothesis on the pathogenesis of schizophrenia:

1. Anyone who is in close contact with schizophrenics is able to demonstrate time and again that healthy life (healthy perception, thinking, judgment, memory, emotion) is preserved side by side with and behind schizophrenic experience. To put it in a slogan one might say: "The healthy man lives on in the schizophrenic." However, "there is also a schizophrenic in the healthy." A form of living that can hardly be differentiated from schizophrenic experience comes to the fore under various circumstances—in dreams, in autistic and archaic thinking, mystic, and in many forms of art, to name but a few examples. But in the schizophrenic a type of experience overrules the existence, and often endangers it, which in the healthy person remains within certain bounds and proceeds under certain prerequisite conditions.

2. In a healthy psychic life we adjust to reality in a manner best designed to permit us to employ our talents and to satisfy our requirements. On the other hand, the schizophrenic neglects this adjustment to reality, and thus the order and harmony of his inner life. A spiritual world develops in the schizophrenic which expresses his own striving and requirements in all their contradictory forms. The psychopathology of the schizophrenic reflects in moving symbolism all the contradictory desires, fears, lusts, sorrows, joys, and contrary experience of man. He has lost sight of the aim to act as a uniform person, uniformly in the fight for existence. What constitutes a healthy personality—its unity, its harmony—is split up.

3. The most severe chronic schizophrenic condition (schizophrenic dementia) differs sharply from the dementia seen in brain diseases. The difference does not only consist in the fact that healthy psychic life is preserved behind the diseased experience (as we have mentioned before), but it is also expressed by the course of the illness. The most severe, chronic schizophrenic conditions can often suddenly improve after many years; in some instances they recover "as if by a miracle." Severe cases of organic dementia, which have lasted for a long time, are never reversible.

4. In general the following rule applies: Patients who are physically ill are not schizophrenics, and schizophrenics are physically healthy. In particular, patients with endocrine diseases are not schizophrenics, and schizophrenics are not endocrinologically ill. (As with all cate-

goric rules and summarized observations, they might be open to some reservations, corrections, and complementary statements, but on the whole I consider them valid.)

5. To date, no pathologic-anatomic or physiologic findings have been discovered which may be interpreted to be the principal cause of genuine, schizophrenic psychoses. Usually physical findings described for schizophrenic patients have not been confirmed by discerning investigators who reinvestigated the facts; in some other patients the criteria described are sequelae rather than causes of the disease, and yet in other instances such findings determined in schizophrenic patients have also been found valid in patients with other diseases or in healthy persons.

6. Schizophrenia runs strongly in certain families. Close relatives of schizophrenics are themselves found to be schizophrenic more often than more remote relatives. But even enzygotic twins of schizophrenics have not been found to be always also schizophrenics. For over 50 years attempts have been made to attribute schizophrenia mainly to one or two mutant genes which would pass from one generation to the next according to Mendel's law. All such attempts to prove that schizophrenia is a hereditary disease subject to simple Mendelian rules have failed.

7. If one gets to know a schizophrenic closely (for instance in the course of analytic therapy) one will find that schizophrenic experience is subjectively felt as a coming to terms with oppressive and contradictory life experiences.

8. Often (though not always) the development of schizophrenia is in close temporal and, presumably, also causal connection with influences from the surroundings. Inappropriate treatment, most particularly and distinctly isolation of the patient, has a negative effect, while some therapeutic measures have a positive influence in some patients and during certain phases. In the course of protracted and psychoanalytic therapy, phases during which the illness is hardly noticeable usually occur (at least transiently).

9. One often has the impression that the conditions of life of the schizophrenic patient prior to the disease have been unfavorable from early childhood on. This is an impression, however, for which we have insufficient proof to date. But we do have significant statistical data indicating that a background of broken families is more

frequent in the parental homes of women who later become schizophrenic than in the general population.

10. In more than half (though not all) of the patients, persons who
will later become schizophrenic are distinguished by personality
traits for which, to date, we have no better comprehensive term than
the word "schizoid." While sexual perversion is no more dominant
in the early history of the schizophrenic patient than it is in the
general population, weak erotic impulses are apparently more frequent among these persons than they are in the average population.
As to physical appearance, we find that irregular proportions between
various physical dimensions occur more often in schizophrenics.

11. There are numerous transitional states between schizophrenic
psychoses and atypical psychoses, in which psychogenic causes obviously play an important role: such psychoses, which must be classified intermediary between schizophrenias and psychogenic psychoses,
are, e.g., many forms of induced insanity, the so-called schizophrenic
reaction, many delusions of grandeur, many acute catatoniform
psychoses in Africans, and many forms of paranoia.

12. Schizophrenia is a frequently occurring disease. As far as we
know its incidence has always remained in the same proportions. (The
probability index for the general population is about one percent.)
On the other hand, the fertility of schizophrenics is much lower than
that of the average population. If schizophrenia were a hereditary
disease, the hereditary factors responsible for the development of
schizophrenic psychoses ought to be reproduced time and again.

What then are the conclusions we can draw from these observations
in regard to the nature and genesis of schizophrenia?

Based on facts and disregarding speculation, we must observe that
no physical basis for schizophrenia has been found to date. Nevertheless, it is clear that the disease often runs in families and that it is
noticeably affected by the patient's life experience. Hence we must
look for the cause of schizophrenia in an inherited predisposition
and in life experience and not in physical, organic conditions. Of
caurse, heredity is always connected with matter, and life experience is always organically bound to the brain. Naturally, in this
sense any disturbance which is based on heredity and life experience
is an organic disturbance. But as a rule the term "organic" is not
intended to be as comprehensive as that, and we usually distinguish
between physical matters and psychologic matters. We call physical

that which is clearly connected with certain physical processes, e.g., progressive paralysis with syphilitic encephalitis, or the mood disturbance in hyperparathyroidism with a certain imbalance in calcium metabolism. Although those processes which we term "psychic experience" of course require a body as a prerequisite for their occurrence, these processes unfold without any noticeable connection with organic processes. Intellectual capacity is based on heredity and life experience, but we cannot relate individual differences and peculiarities to any definitive anatomic or functional physical conditions. As far as we are able to perceive them, the brain and metabolism of men with varying life experiences and different, inborn intelligence are the same. If we proclaim that schizophrenia has no discernible physical basis, we mean that it is "purely psychic," in the same sense as neurotic and most psychopathic trends (and, for that matter, healthy personality development) are purely psychic. Of course, everything purely psychic is also rooted in the body and multifaceted interrelations, few of which are known to us exist.

We have no grounds, however, to seek the basis of schizophrenia in an inborn error of metabolism. First of all, none has been found despite painstaking research; and secondly, all known inborn errors of metabolism, far from resulting in schizophrenia, are responsible for other psychic disturbances, e.g., above all, feeblemindedness and epilepsy.

What then are the hereditary prerequisites for the development of schizophrenia? It has now become highly improbable that they can be attributed to one or two genes altered by mutation. No Mendelian heredity has been established for schizophrenia. Furthermore, in view of the high incidence of schizophrenia and the low rate of fertility of schizophrenics, we would have to assume such a high rate of mutation as has never been observed anywhere else. But we can assume that schizophrenias are based on multiple inherited tendencies. Are we then dealing with numerous, unfavorable, mutant, disease-producing genes? Or, can healthy genes in an unfavorable combination perhaps yield the prerequisites for the development of schizophrenia? In part, posing this question is superfluous. Up to a point it is entirely arbitrary whether we speak of polygenic or disharmonious dispositions, when most genes which—in combination—may predispose an individual for a disease, may—in a different genic environment—contribute to healthy development. But theoretically there is, nevertheless, a difference between the concept of polygenic predisposition towards disease, on the one hand, and disturbed harmony in tendencies which are basically healthy, on the other, if we formulate it as follows: The multiple genes which, in combination, predispose a subject towards schizophrenia are genes where unfavorable mutation has taken place. However, we have absolutely no valid indications which imply that genes altered by mutation might result in schizophrenia. By contrast, as far as we know to date, mutant genes which affect psychic life lead to feeble-mindedness or epilepsy.

Conversely, many observations are much more readily reconcilable with the idea that a lack of compatibility, an absence of harmony between inherited psychic characteristics of development, may account for the hereditary disposition towards schizophrenia. This assumption readily explains why the incidence of schizophrenia has—to our knowledge—remained constant in spite of the low rate of fertility among schizophrenics. It also fits in much better than the mutation hypothesis with the observation that schizophrenia is found in all the peoples of the world.

We must also note, however, that a predisposition for schizophrenia, as we now know it, consists essentially of disharmonious characteristics. The schizoid individual finds it difficult to adjust uniformly and to balance the contradictions in his own being. Physical schizophrenic disposition consists primarily in unharmonious proportions between various parts of the body.

We must also consider though that the unity of the personality is by no means a predetermined, unalterable fact. Developmental psychology has taught us quite clearly that the ego, the personality, develops slowly. A fully structured, uniform personality develops from a sum of inborn reactions and developmental dispositions. The result should be a hierarchy of divergent tendencies, adjusted to life experience. Isolated contradictions are basic to the tragic development of healthy persons and to neurotic development. Nevertheless, the personality is preserved as a total uniform structure. But in schizophrenic experience this unity is lost. Numerous, deep seated conflicts are no longer resolved. Normal psychology, neuroses, and, ultimately in a very special measure, our knowledge of schizophrenia teach us that the ego, the personality as a uniform structure, is constantly in danger; child psychology has shown us that during the first years of life the child must fumblingly grope for this unity on the basis of his experience. Should we really assume that inborn psychic reactions and developmental dispositions must always fit equally readily and harmoniously into a unified whole? Does not experience alone already suggest that inadequate matches, disharmonious inborn psychic developmental dispositions may indeed occur? And, if they do occur we must expect them most often as inborn dispositions, especially in schizophrenics who are characterized by a high degree of disintegration of the entire uniform personality.

No psychogenetic theory of schizophrenia can dispense with the assumption of hereditary disposition. One of the reasons is that there are no psychotraumatic situations in the prehistory of a schizophrenic which have not been experienced equally by numerous other people, who did not become schizophrenic.

Nor is there any hypothesis on hereditary schizophrenia that could dispense with the assumption that life experiences provide additional causes. The importance of acquired causes is evidenced, among other things, by the fact that by no means do all enzygotic twins of schizophrenics also develop into schizophrenics. Moreover, the clinician, unlike the genetic research worker, is daily confronted by the experience that the condition of schizophrenic patients may improve or deteriorate considerably as a result of facts obviously connected with the development in the patient's human environment. With the best intentions it is utterly impossible to draw any sharp lines between psychoses where psychogenia is apparent, psychoses where psychogenia is probable, and pure schizophrenias.

If disharmonious developmental dispositions form the hereditary basis of schizophrenia, i.e. of the disease characterized by awesome disharmonies of psychic life, it is only natural that we should seek the essential psychotraumatic background of the disease in disharmonious life experience.

To date, we have no proof that this assumption is correct and such proof is difficult to come by. But there is also nothing to disprove it and we have significant indications that there may be substance to this conjecture: Margareth Singer, Lyman Wynne, and others have collected a vast amount of data which would imply that unclear, ambiguous, contradictory thought processes and manners of expression are a quality of the parents of schizophrenics. It is highly probable that there is a connection between the confused intellectual personality of the parents of schizophrenic patients and the pathogenesis of this disease in their children. Lidz, Alanen, and other authors have shown that sex roles and the proper place of different generations are indistinct and ambiguous in the families from which schizophrenics originate. And, indeed, we can often observe the conflicting composure of the schizophrenic in regard to his own sex role or place in the scheme of generations. An extraordinary amount of contradictory and conflicting experiences in the early history of the schizophrenic patient has also come to light in my own practical experience. For instance, there are patients who as children assumed a different intellectual talent and other interests than those the parents had assumed, so that their striving went off in different directions from those their parents had expected and approved. Again in other patients the life ideals of mother, stepmother, and father were in conflict.

Even more important than these experiences is what the schizophrenics themselves say about these inner conflicts, splits, and contradictions. They experience them as the necessary consequence of contradictory, conflicting life experiences which they are unable to surmount.

Modern schizophrenia research has also made it possible for us to gain some insight into the character of the interplay between inherited disposition towards disease and dangerous life experiences. Earlier, research workers had assumed that the inherited tendency could be held in check, and they often viewed the inherited essence of a human being and his life experiences as independent of one another. But since we have begun to observe the psychopathologic development of schizophrenics we have learned that the basic nature of the patient and his life experiences are closely interrelated. The same holds true for a person's healthy development: His life experience, and above all his relations to other people are not only molded by external circumstances but, to a large extent, by himself. Time and again we note that there are warped and confused human relationships in the prehistory of patients who later become schizophrenics.If we ask ourselves whether he himself was responsible for the trouble, or whether it was because of unfavorable circumstances or the fault of his fellow creatures, or both, we usually find it difficult to come to any conclusions. Just as the patient has provoked unfavorable developments in his relationships, so have these unfavorable developments in return affected him. It is rarely possible to pinpoint which was the primary cause, hence we must assume that the question was inappropriately put in the first place. The basic nature of the patient and his human relationships have become warped jointly by rubbing against one another.

If we take into consideration what we now know about schizophrenia, and try to refrain from proclaiming and expounding on that which we do not know, we can now describe the nature and essence of schizophrenic psychoses—in my opinion—approximately as the following:

Schizophrenic disease develops as a result of an interrelation between unfavorable, disharmonious inherited psychic reactions and developmental dispositions, and unfavorable and disharmonious life experience. No direct physical background for this development has been discovered, just as there is no such organic basis in neuroses or psychopathic development, nor in the differentiation of unique personalities of those persons who are healthy.

The question has been asked whether, in view of the fact that, to date, neurotic and healthy personality development have also been attributed largely to inborn, psychic developmental dispositions and life experience, is schizophrenia then nothing else but a neurosis? No, it is a psychosis, not a neurosis! But its history of development need not be sought in spheres entirely different from those basic to neuroses. It does not differ in its principal pathogenesis, but rather sharply in its result. The schizophrenic transcends into an autistic world, while the neurotic continues to dwell in the world of the sane, merely getting lost in some isolated spheres of life.

The strongest support for our sketchy concept of schizophrenia comes from our therapeutic experience. In the treatment of schizophrenics we have used, successfully, the same forces which develop the personality, self-consciousness, and the ego in childhood: active human mutual participation and the surprise and shock up to a degree where it endangers the very existence. Indeed, from a purely empirical point of view, the principle of active communal participation has proven the most successful therapeutic element in the treatment of schizophrenics. Such communal participation develops from diverse circumstances: work therapy, group therapy, and individual psychotherapy, so-called "moralistic therapy" (Baruk), as well as many other methods. As modern developmental psychology has shown, the decisive force in the development of each personality is the active communal participation with the mother, the parental family, and other human beings.

The second principle of successful therapy for schizophrenic patients consists in surprise and shock (by abrupt analytic interpretation, sudden shouldering of responsibility, unannounced transfers, and shock therapy). Shock and danger, to the very essence of existence, also stimulate the healthy person to gather his wits and are compelling forces—even in normal development—for an individual to comport himself uniformly and direct all his attention to the fight for existence.

A third principle of schizophrenic therapy consists in reassurance (by contact, encouragement, and neuroleptics). In many instances it is possible to bring about active communal participation without preceding sedation. Reassuring and calming the highly excited patient is as important in the therapy of the schizophrenic as calm and consideration are for the child who needs these influences as much as he needs stimulation.

In summary, based on what we have outlined above (and much that still remains to be said), we can formulate the genesis and nature of schizophrenia as follows:

Schizophrenia is a disease which develops on the basis of disharmonious life experience. Just as an essentially disharmonious human being will mold his surroundings in a disharmonious pattern, so will a disharmonious environment intensify the inborn, internal disharmonies. Schizophrenic psychosis, as such, consists of a disharmonious personality, an overflowing of psychic life, which is not uniformly directed towards its environment, but rather produces images of the world which reflect its own inner strife. In the therapy of schizophrenia we make use of the same forces which develop the personality of the healthy person towards oneness.

It is unlikely that these concepts embrace the ultimate truth on schizophrenia. Perhaps important new discoveries will compel us to change these concepts in the future. I make no claim that the hypothesis I have presented has final validity. It is merely a modest attempt to summarize the insight we have gained to date, and represents only a preliminary hypothesis on the nature and pathogenesis of schizophrenia, based on clinical experience and not on speculation.

If such hypotheses have any value at all nowadays, it is this: They force us to take the empirical therapeutic experience in the treatment of schizophrenics seriously. This is not a symptomatic, superficial therapy for want of overall, causal therapy. We are justified in taking it seriously, and society should make more support available for it than is the case to date in most countries.

Lastly, the hypothesis outlined above poses a new task for our research. We should pay more attention to the multiplicity of predispositions than we did in the past, rather than expect a single or, at most, a few decisive causes; for it is the interaction between those diverse trends which will ultimately result in what are termed schizophrenic psychoses.

2

Research in Schizophrenia

WILLIAM MALAMUD, M.D.

Director, Program of Research in Schizophrenia
Scottish Rite Northern Jurisdiction, U.S.A.

The scope of this article, as suggested by its title, quite justifiably might be considered inordinately ambitious. However, this paper is not intended as a comprehensive presentation of the nature and results of all current studies; instead, what is brought before you here is the trend of present research in psychiatry, particularly in schizophrenia.

In this field, as in medicine in general, there has always been a strong, almost compelling tendency for research to proceed in terms of patterns or trends. On rare occasions throughout history, there have been lone investigations (and investigators) that have produced results which are so objectively valid and fundamentally true that they become accepted, in toto, as permanent components of the total body of medical knowledge, but this is the exception in research; by far, most knowledge has been gleaned from the laborious pursuit of trends, with each new study influencing the course of the trend by serving to reinforce or contradict the theoretical basis of work that has prompted and preceded it.

Many trends have been abandoned because further studies have failed to bear out the findings of the initial investigation on which they were based. Many other trends have been abandoned because of a lack of adequate methodology to substantiate essentially sound principles, and these have often been reintroduced as methodology has improved and new avenues of approach have opened up.

Thus, present trends in research in schizophrenia will be considered here in terms of their emergence, their relation to research in the past, their present status, and the problems which tend to aid or impede their progress.

16

Schizophrenia is still the number one problem in psychiatry, being the most prevalent in terms of incidence, the most devastating in its effects, the most ill defined in concept, and the least understood, in terms of its nature, causes, course, and outcome. The global nature of the impact of schizophrenia on personality functions, furthermore, renders any new knowledge of this disease potentially applicable to practically all other psychopathologic disturbances.

When taking stock of the scientific contributions made throughout the history of research in psychiatry in general, and schizophrenia in particular, the enormous increase in quantity, scope, and quality of this work during the last two or three decades, as compared with any other period in the past, is profoundly impressive. There are even those who are of the opinion that most of the scientifically adequate and reliable investigative work in this field has been contributed since the Second World War. It is essential to remember, however, that some important research has been conducted in various periods in the past, and that some of its results have served as precursors to present day investigations. Just where the starting point of systematic investigation in this field should be placed is largely a matter of personal interests and experiences. Thus, one could start with the work of Benjamin Rush, and his theory that mental diseases are due to disturbances in cerebral circulation; or one might date all worthwhile investigation from the time of the critical epidemiologic studies of Pliny Earle and his attempts to establish the real factors involved in the "cult of curability." Similarly, one could start with the neuropathologic studies of Nissl and Alzeheimer, and their followers, or with Kretschmer's introduction of the theory of constitutional types, as it related to the concept of constitution and heredity in general.

The concept of dynamics introduced by psychoanalysis, the holistic concept of psychobiology, and other concepts less well known, have provided bases for research of greater or lesser impact. Even during my own professional experience, which is now closely approaching the half-century mark, I have seen results of research corroborated or disproved, some theories falling by the wayside, others serving as forerunners of some present day investigative work. I started my residency in psychiatry about the time when Kirby and Kopeloff were in the midst of their investigation of the validity of the focal infection theory. I participated for a time in the work of the neuroendocrine program in Worcester, which was initiated in the late twenties. At about that time, the shock therapies and lobotomy were introduced, and the overly enthusiastic reports by some of the protagonists of these methods, while perhaps somewhat less than objective, did serve to spur a considerable amount of investigation, both applied and basic. A number of other areas of psychiatric research were newly opened up during that era, or were approached with new purposefulness, which was reflected in an impressive increase in research activity in that period. These included studies of the dynamics of child behavior and its importance to the understanding of personality disturbances in adults as well as children; the impact of the psychoanalytic theory of the dynamics of human development and psychopathologic processes; studies on sociopsychopathology by Sullivan; the psychobiologic approach of Adolph Meyer; the development of the concept of psychosomatics, and more. Contribution in these areas, which began in the early years of this century or in the later nineteenth century, all initiated trends in investigation, and many are still being pursued fruitfully and further explored today.

Nevertheless, until quite recently, psychiatric research has lagged behind the other medical disciplines, and despite present acceleration, it is both thought-provoking and prudent to question what factors caused this earlier lag, and to consider whether it is possible that some of these factors persist, still acting as unrecognized deterrents to progress.

Some of the most important factors responsible for this earlier paucity of psychiatric research can be categorized as follows:

1. The determined search for a single cause and quick remedy, as a main motivating stimulus, doomed many research programs to failure before they began. Considering the overwhelming nature of the conditions that faced earlier psychiatrists, this approach is understandable. Hospital populations were increasing at an alarming rate, and the victims of mental illness, particularly those with schizophrenia, presented an unyielding chronicity for which no form of effective rational treatment had yet been discovered. It is no wonder, therefore, that any achievement of symptomatic improvement, induced empirically, or by serendipity, was likely to have its efficacy exaggerated. Such a climate provided fertile ground for the development of spurious theories of the mechanisms or the pathologic factors involved.

2. Lack of adequate research methods made it difficult to conduct

reliable studies; findings so attained defied interdisciplinary correlation. This difficulty was particularly crippling in the attempts to discern relationships between biologic and psychosocial phenomena, for even in those instances where a positive correlation seemed obvious, the nature and extent of the association could not be determined because of the lack of tests or criteria which were equally valid, common or even logically relevant to both.

3. Psychiatrists tended to isolate themselves from other professional and scientific workers, particularly up to the turn of the century, but to some extent even after that. With a few notable exceptions, psychiatrists limited themselves to their own field, to carry on their work, be it clinical or investigative, by themselves. The result, of course, was a restriction of the concept of the personality and its disorders, and a failure to take into consideration the important role of the interdependence of psychologic and physiologic factors in determining behavior in toto. Needless to add, this divorcement was a two-way process, involving both sides in this schism. It has only been recognized within very recent years that the human being must be considered as a whole, if we are to understand his behavior in health or disease.

4. The failure to recognize disease as a dynamic process rather than a pathologic state seemed to plague psychiatric investigation longer than it continued to handicap research in other areas. In a way, it must be said that man has always known that disease has an onset, a course, and an end, and to that extent it is a process. In the past, however, this process was viewed quite rudimentarily as a summation of a series of states, the appreciation of any one of which could be made on the basis of a cross section at any given time. This was especially evident in the accepted pathologic anatomy of the past, when the pathologic state was considered by most workers to be a sort of discrete entity in itself. It was only at about the turn of the century that a number of scientists from various disciplines independently developed the concept of a dynamic process of disease, and set the trend toward present thinking. Freud, in psychopathology, Krehl, in medicine, and a number of others described such a dynamic process in terms of ongoing changes in the whole individual.

5. The nebulousness of the definition of schizophrenia has handicapped research into this disease entity. It would seem logical to expect that if we are to undertake a discussion of research in schizophrenia,

we must start out with a clear definition of what we mean by schizo-phrenia, and yet it appears that while we are all familiar with the phenomenology of its features and even, in most cases, agree on the diagnosis, a good deal of fogginess still persists when we attempt to define it.

There is no question but that the patient who was described by Morel in 1860 as having "dementia praecox" would have been diag-nosed as schizophrenic by most clinicians today, even if many would question the theory that Morel advanced in regard to the cause of this illness. Furthermore, a comprehensive description of precisely what we are dealing with in schizophrenia has remained elusive, de-spite the contributions of Hecker, Kahlbaum, Wernicke, Kraepelin, Bleuler, and others, who have so diligently attempted to sharpen the definition of this condition as a clinical entity in a manner that could be generally accepted, agreed upon, and understood. There is no question about the fact that schizophrenia is a disease entity, with certain recognizable characteristics of its own, because today, just as years ago, the same patients who are diagnosed as being schizophrenic by one experienced psychiatrist will be so diagnosed by any number of others of equal experience, with the rate of concurrence being very high. Yet, it remains very difficult to state in objective terms what it is that characterizes this disease process and differentiates it from others. As a result of this discouraging elusiveness, there have been differences of opinion with regard to the range of psychopathology that should be included as schizophrenic. There are those, for instance, who limit the diagnosis of true schizophrenia to the narrow confines of a central type of process, defining all others as "schizophrenialike." Then there are distinctions made between process versus reactive types, schizo-affective forms, pseudoneurotic, and more. It is not hard to understand the difficulty of arriving at any kind of generally acceptable conclusions regarding the pathology and, particularly, the etiology, of a process so ill defined and widely scattered.

Much of the progress of research that has been achieved, partic-ularly in recent years, was made possible by the solution of some of these problems which had been deterrents in the past. Some still exist and will have to be dealt with through the introduction of further changes.

Certainly, few still cling to the notion of a single cause and the companion hope that, once this causative agent or mechanism has been revealed, a "blanket," all-encompassing therapeutic maneuver can be perceived which will provide quick and curative remedial results.

Also, it can no longer be said that the psychiatrist, and particularly the psychiatrist-investigator, still isolates himself from other scientists and the findings of other branches of medical science. Nor is he isolated by his fellow workers in other fields today. A former aura of aloof detachment that characterized workers on both sides of this once unbridgeable schism has been replaced by attitudes that vary all the way from avid, open-minded interest, and an eagerness to learn from one another, to a staid and cautious, almost reluctant willingness to listen, at least, to the proponents of ideas born of other disciplines of medical science. The fellowship of medicine which encompasses *all* of the healing arts is overtaking and replacing the former relationship which extended only to the peripheries of the specialized sciences.

Nonetheless, in examining all three of the remaining deterrents that handicapped investigators of the past, we find that much still remains to be accomplished.

While it is true that over the years there has been a progressive improvement in methods of research, there is still a definite need for further refinements, particularly for methods suitable for interdisciplinary or transdisciplinary research.

In a general sense, the concept of disease being a dynamic process has been widely accepted, but in its practical application, both experimental and clinical, a number of fundamental issues have not received the attention they deserve. This is the case, for instance, with regard to investigations of etiology. We still think in terms of original causes as the only important determinants, all others being secondary or contributory, failing to recognize the fact that in the course of the process, the effects of original causes may in their turn become the causes of disturbances which may prove to be more serious than the original ones.

PRESENT STATUS OF RESEARCH

Despite problems unresolved, handicaps still operant, and a lack of total concurrence of opinion, a full understanding, or even an acceptable clear definition of the enemy we are fighting, research delving into the problem of schizophrenia continues to forge ahead.

Upon surveying the present status of research, the rate as well as the substance of recent progress has been so great that this acceleration almost appears to have taken place abruptly on the basis of some particular development that served to introduce the change. A closer analysis, however, shows this to have been a gradual process, rather than a sudden emergence of insight. A number of important investigations that are being conducted at the present time can be seen as a broadening of scope of some studies that were started some years ago. The early 1930s witnessed a very definite increase in research activity in psychiatry in general, and schizophrenia in particular. Of particular importance was the gradual influx of research techniques from related fields such as biochemistry, physiology, the social sciences, psychology, and psychopathology. There is a broad increase in the scope of the field, taking in all of the clinical and basic sciences relevant to this disease. Perhaps the best way of indicating some aspects of this progress is to discuss them in terms of trends that are particularly prominent in this field today.

PRESENT TRENDS

Three trends stand out as especially significant, and cover a good deal of the work that is being conducted. These include investigations in the area of (1) genetics, as related to environmental factors; (2) the individual in his ecologic setting; and (3) the correlation between the psychic and somatic aspects of personality functions.

Nature or Nurture

The role played by heredity in determining human behavior in general, and abnormal behavior in particular, has occupied the mind of man in the course of his entire history. The early theories, and especially popular notions that mental disease is the result of hereditary factors only, and that the development of the disease in an individual should be regarded as an expression of the inevitable destiny of that person, have given rise to many inquiries over the years, eventually leading to the formulation of three possible hypotheses: (1) that mental diseases are due entirely or, at least, primarily to inherited factors and that environmental stress may, at most, affect the form but not the essence of the disease; (2) that environmental stress and strain, in the form of physical or sociopsychologic trauma, is the primary factor in determining the adjustment or maladjustment of the person, as expressed in the concept that the person starts life as a *tabula rasa* on which environment and experience inscribe the ultimate behavioral characteristics; (3) most present day workers in this area, however, are of the opinion that behavior is a result of the interaction between the person's hereditary or constitutional anlage and the environment to which he has had to adjust. Anlage provides patterns and tools which the person uses in coping with problems he encounters, and when the former are deficient, or the latter presents overwhelming problems (or both), his ability to cope in a healthy, productive manner is exceeded and maladjustment results.

The earlier studies in this area simply consisted of geneologic surveys of the families of mentally ill persons for the purpose of finding out whether the familial incidence of mental illness was significantly greater than it was in the average background of normal persons. This method was in vogue for a long time, but is infrequently used today, except for the purpose of obtaining supportive data. A definite improvement in methodology was the development of the studies of twins in which the rate of concordance in monozygotic and dizygotic twins and nontwin siblings was investigated. Despite the fact that these studies yielded more adequate, accurate, and objective data, they were still not entirely conclusive because they failed to remove the possible influence of certain environmental factors. In the first place, although concordance in the identical twins was definitely more frequent than in nonidentical twin pairs, there still were some identical twins which were discordant, and in order to find the reason for that, it became necessary to look for factors other than those of heredity which might have been important to the pathologic development of a single member of an identical pair. Discordance in the development of identical twins posed the question that since a monozygotic twin pair were more likely to have a similar hereditary anlage than others, had there been a difference in the developmental environment of these twins of sufficient importance to account for their lack of concordance? More recently, the biologic as well as psychologic nature of the hereditary factors is being scrutinized more closely.

The idea that the environmental stress of early childhood may play an important role in the development of mental illness in later years has been emphasized for a long time, but the attempts to test the validity of this concept have met with varying degrees of success, depending upon the methodology used. In attempting to probe the childhoods of the adult subjects under scrutiny, many earlier studies depended largely on histories obtained from these same patients and their relatives, although it is obvious that little objective, scientifically valid data could be hoped for from such a source. The more recent studies in this field have tried to avoid this source of error by studying children from birth onward, recording the objective findings of separate observers. This, obviously, is a much more dependable, but time-consuming, method of approach; but in addition to the advantage of being more reliable and objective, such a plan of study has a "built-in" source of controls, since obviously most of its subjects can be expected to develop normally, with these providing adequate controls for the number who later prove to be abnormal. Over the years, the methods utilized in this approach have been progressively refined and rendered more reliable, and new ones have been introduced.

Studies in this area, furthermore, have been directed toward the nature of the genetic factor which serves as the predisposing agent. Is it an inborn metabolic error? Is it some endocrine disturbance? Is it some enzyme deficiency, or is it some peculiar characteristic of the nervous system, central or sympathetic? Recent progress has made it possible to gain a better understanding of the nature and function of genetic factors and the role they play in determining human behavior, and the nature vs. nurture dichotomy will most probably not be resolved in the form of an "either/or" answer, but in terms of a type of interaction of the two.

The Person and His Ecologic Setting

Events are expressions of an ongoing process, rather than isolated states, and they are manifestations of whole settings, including the individual and his environment.

To understand any act of behavior or event in experience, it is essential to obtain valid data regarding the past, as well as the present, of the individual as well as of his former and present ecologic setting. There is no doubt today that it is very important to obtain from the individual an account of his experiences, particularly during the formative years, from the standpoint of treatment and the evaluation of his present condition. This, however, is primarily important in terms of his interpretation of events; what they meant (and mean) to him form the basis of his present attitudes.

Beside the reactions of the individual, as well as others in the setting, in terms of feelings and attitudes as they experienced them at that time, general ecologic factors may have important bearing, such as sounds, movements, states of discomfort, threatening or reassuring stimuli, crowding or isolation, etc. The reactions, as observed objectively or reported by the subject, are the result of an interrelationship of the individual, inseparable from his unique ecology, which has shaped him, and which he has also altered.

Correlation Between Psychic and Somatic Aspects

One of the most persistent problems throughout the years, and one which still confronts us today, is the failure to resolve the schism inherent in the concept of body-mind dualism.

Entry into the field of psychiatric research of some of the best minds in the biologic sciences, and the interest among psychiatrists in the contributions made by these workers, have at least helped to improve communication, widening horizons on both sides. This has led to a series of investigations of correlates between the biologic and behavioral aspects of the phenomena of personality disorders.

A good example of the results of research along these lines is afforded by recent reports of pathologic findings in the blood plasma constituents of schizophrenic patients. These reports, although not identical, have been published by a number of laboratories during the last decade. Some of the workers have reported the manifestation of transient psychoticlike behavior following the introduction of concentrated amounts of this factor into the blood stream of normal organisms. Others have reported indications of a genetic origin of these abnormalities. Still others have investigated the possibility of the existence of an antagonist to this factor which could serve as an inhibitor of its production and level of concentration. This aspect of research may be designated, for want of a better term, as the "psychosomatic" character of the problem of schizophrenia.

Many questions remain to be answered, and each new study opens newer avenues to pursue. The study of correlations between psychic and physical pathologic phenomena has barely begun to scratch the surface. Certainly, attempts to tie these aspects together have not always succeeded in producing universally acceptable results, but it is also possible that the schism has been perpetuated more by differences in the points of view of proponents of various solutions than by differences inherent in the problem itself.

3

Early Infantile Autism Revisited

LEO KANNER, M.D.

Professor Emeritus, Johns Hopkins U. School of Medicine

The year 1968 marks the first quarter-century anniversary of a publication in which this author reported a pattern of child behavior which had not previously been considered in its striking uniqueness. The paper, appearing in 1943 in the now extinct journal, *The Nervous Child*, dealt in some detail with 11 children (eight boys and three girls) who presented a combination of extreme aloneness from the beginning of life and an anxiously obsessive insistence on the preservation of sameness (1). In searching for an appropriate designation, I decided, after much groping, on the term "early infantile autism," which described time of the first manifestations and accentuated the children's limited accessibility. Beyond the descriptive nosographic account, I ventured this opinion: *We must assume that these children have come into the world with an innate inability to form the usual, biologically-provided affective contact with people, just as other children come into the world with innate physical and intellectual handicaps. . . . Here, we seem to have pure-culture examples of inborn autistic disturbances of affective contact.*

From the start I was greatly impressed with one observation which stood out prominently: The parents of these patients were, for the most part, strongly preoccupied with abstractions of a scientific, literary, or artistic nature, and limited in genuine interest in people. As time went on and more autistic children were studied, the coincidence of infantile autism and the parents' mechanized form of living was really startling. This was confirmed by many other observers. I noted then, however: *These children's aloneness from the beginning*

27

of life makes it difficult to attribute the whole picture exclusively to the type of early parental relationships that they have experienced.

At no time have I pointed to the parents as the primary, postnatal sources of pathogenicity.

The publication of the case findings of the first 11 patients was prompted merely by a wish to communicate to my colleagues a number of experiences for which I could find no reference in the literature. It did not, and could not, occur to me at the time that we were on the threshold of creating, unexpectedly and unintentionally, a great deal of excitement in the field of child psychiatry. This was, in fact, a piece of serendipity, an unpremeditated "discovery" which was not the result of a specific search. Of course, I was interested in the peculiarities of the illness; more such children came to my attention, and I made and reported several studies on the irrelevant and metaphoric language of some of these patients, on their conception of wholes and parts, and on their family backgrounds. In 1949, these findings and assumptions were cautiously summarized in a paper entitled, "Problems of Nosology and Psychodynamics of Early Infantile Autism" (2).

In retrospect, the brief history of infantile autism can be separated into three consecutive phases:

While the case reports published in 1943 almost immediately received the attention of the profession, it took some time before similar observations could be made and communicated. The earliest reports by other authors dealing with the issue did not appear for several years.

This state of affairs changed abruptly in 1951. No fewer than 52 articles and one book, concerned specifically with this subject, appeared between then and 1959. The first European confirmations of the existence of the syndrome came in 1952 from van Krevelen in Holland, and from Stern in France (3, 4).

As these reports began to accrue, it became apparent that while the majority of the Europeans were satisfied with a sharp delineation of infantile autism as a specific illness *sui generis,* there was a tendency in this country to view it as a developmental anomaly ascribed exclusively to maternal emotional determinants. Moreover, it became a habit to dilute the original concept of infantile autism by diagnosing it in many disparate conditions which showed one or another isolated symptom found as a feature of the overall syndrome. Almost overnight this country seemed to be populated by a multitude of autistic children, and this trend began to become noticeable overseas as well. Mentally defective children who displayed bizarre behavior were promptly labeled autistic and, in accordance with preconceived notions, both parents were urged to undergo protracted psychotherapy in addition to treatment directed toward the defective child's own supposedly underlying emotional problem. By 1953, van Krevelen became impatient with the confused and confusing use of the term infantile autism as a slogan, indiscriminately applied, with cavalier abandonment of the criteria which had been outlined rather succinctly and unmistakably from the beginning. He warned against the prevailing "abuse of the diagnosis of autism," declaring that it "threatens to become a fashion" (5). A little slower to anger, I made a similar plea for the acknowledgment of the specificity of the illness and for adherence to the established criteria at the International Psychiatric Congress in Zurich in 1957 (6).

By 1960, the fashion deplored by van Krevelen had gradually subsided. This was perhaps caused in part by the fact that those who go in for the summary adoption of diagnostic clichés found another handy label for a variety of abnormalities. Instead of the many "autistic" children who are not autistic, we have now the ever-ready rubber stamp of "brain-damage." While this is also regrettable, it has at least driven the diagnostic faddists to jump onto another bandwagon, and has left the serious study of autism to those pledged to diagnostic accuracy. Hence, it has now become easier to single out properly designated cases; true autism is now less apt to be lost in the shuffle of a peculiarly miscellaneous deck which could only serve to obscure an investigation of the pathognomonic characteristics of this illness. Indeed, in the past few years the diagnoses made have been more uniformly reliable and the discussion has been considerably less obfuscated by the smuggling in of irrelevant case material.

By now, thanks to several efforts at diagnostic refinement, the existence of the syndrome, as such, has been universally acknowledged. Several books and hundreds of articles attest to the interest which it has aroused in many quarters, especially on this continent, in Western and Central Europe, and in Japan, but there is still much speculation and understandable confusion concerning etiology and therapy. Notions expounded on this subject have ranged all the way from the assumption of basic organicity to the idea proffered recently which ascribes the illness to the effects of profound parental psychopathology. There are conflicting opinions about the relation between autism and childhood schizophrenia. The concept of operant conditioning occasionally has been misapplied; in precipitous zeal, this approach to therapy has been championed as a foregone success on the basis of what are, in fact, fragmentary attainments. Various groups have exhibited an attitude of monopolistic ownership of anything pertaining to autism and from time to time have awed the lay press with "evidence" of miraculous-sounding cures.

Fortunately, parents in this and a few other countries have recently banded together into special associations, and these groups are making an organized effort to obtain whatever clarification is possible at this time about the nature and prognosis of their children's autism.

Where, then, do we stand at present with regard to our knowledge of early infantile autism? What progress has been made since the first report 25 years ago? What lies ahead of us in the near future? Here are a few points for consideration:

The existence of early infantile autism is generally accepted as a syndrome known to have specific and typical symptomatology and well-defined diagnostic criteria, but it matters little whether autism be regarded as a form of schizophrenia or looked upon as a disease *sui generis*. Since Bleuler's (7) courageous—and as time has proved, correct—refusal to view schizophrenia as a disease entity, and his insistence that there is a "group of schizophrenias," there should be no quarrel with those who wish to retain for autism a place within the "group." Nor should there be any objection to those who would maintain that "Kanner's syndrome" is so clearly delineated that it stands apart in its uniqueness. The issue is more semantic than basic. The illness has been, in either case, split off from the cluster of "the schizophrenias" and has been singled out for investigation of its specific features; it has (and is dealt with by most authors as having) an identity of its own.

It is recognized by all observers, except for the dwindling number of those impeded by doctrinaire allegiances, that autism is not primarily an acquired, or "man-made" disease. The fact that many of the parents are rather detached people has been confirmed frequently enough, but this observation cannot be translated summarily into a direct cause-and-effect etiologic relationship, an assumption sometimes ascribed to me via pathways of gross misquotation. Making parents feel guilty of responsibility for their child's autism is not only erroneous, but cruelly adds insult to injury.

Considerable research has so far failed to produce evidence of any consistent neurologic, metabolic, or chromosomal pathology which can be connected with the origin of autism. Infantile autism is a relatively rare illness, hence, many pediatricians and psychiatrists have had little opportunity to become acquainted with it, and diagnostic uncertainties are to be expected. Even the most experienced know that in some instances differential diagnosis may present difficulties, but it is hoped that there are at least a few professionals in each population center who are familiar with the conditions with which autism could be confused. There are still parents driven to despair by the differing "diagnoses" given out by the various physicians consulted: On the one hand, children who are severely retarded, children with Heller's disease, or who are aphasic, have been miscalled "autistic"; on the other hand, autistic children have been miscalled mentally retarded or aphasic. Valid diagnostic criteria are now available (and have been since 1943), and adherence to these is important. We are still in the dark about the true etiology; it is one thing to speculate about "impairment of the reticular formation" and to philosophize about its role by inference, analogy, and deduction, and still another to have established concrete facts.

The futility of such speculation is illustrated by a recent publication, *The Empty Fortress* (8), published in 1967. Its intrepid dust jacket promised the reader that it "sheds new light on the nature, origin and treatment of infantile autism," but the author of the book, being perhaps somewhat more hampered by actual fact than the author of the dust jacket, felt called upon to employ such qualifications as "maybe," "perhaps," "probably," "possibly," "as if," "as it were," 'seemed to," "suggests," 146 times in 48 pages of the report of the first case, and he cautions his readers further within the text, "This, like other interpretations of Laurie's behavior, is highly speculative. . . ."

Realistically, we must at present accept the fact that our knowledge of the etiology of autism is still extremely limited, and when facts are not available, there is, to be sure, room for theory and hypothesis which lend themselves to sober validation; modesty, however, and the discipline integral to all proper scientific investigation, should protect us from lapses in which we are moved to forget that, however tempting, a theory, unproved, is only that.

This modesty, humility and caution must be applied to therapy as well as to etiology, and this is the keynote at certain centers where efforts continue to be made, consistently and patiently, to help these children find their way into a world which is threatening to them. Other techniques are also being practiced which are founded on theories which have been so dogmatically pronounced and pursued that one must wonder if the earnest "believers" do not hope to elevate their speculative philosophy to the realm of proven fact by dint of pure zeal and enthusiasm—but so far, no better results have been obtained with these theoretically-based techniques than have been obtained with the calm, persistent, non-spectacular attempts to wean the autistic child away from his self-isolation.

This is where we stand at present, approximately 25 years after the first report of 11 autistic children. Much research, much curiosity, are still needed, but so, also, is the kind of sobriety which shies away from fancy-born, pseudo-scientific and premature shouts of *Eureka!*

REFERENCES

1. KANNER, L., *The Nervous Child*, 2:217-250, 1943.
2. KANNER, L., *Amer. J. Orthopsychiat.*, 19:416-426, 1949.
3. VAN KREVELEN, D. A., *Z. Kinderpsychiat.*, 19:91-97, 1952.
4. STERN, E., *Arch. Franc. Pediat.*, 9:157-164, 1952.
5. VAN KREVELEN, D. A., *Acta Neurol. Belg.*, 54:207-212, 1954.
6. KANNER, L., *Rev. Psychiat. Infant.*, 25:108-113, 1958.
7. BLEULER, E., *Dementia Praecox or the Group of Schizophrenias*, International University Press, New York, 1950.
8. BETTELHEIM, B., *The Empty Fortress: Infantile Autism and the Birth of the Self*, The Free Press, New York, 1967.

4

The Crisis of Middle Age

JUDD MARMOR, M.D.

Director, Divisions of Psychiatry, Cedars-Sinai Medical Center
Clinical Professor of Psychiatry, U. of California at Los Angeles

In recent years, the concept of crisis has occupied an increasingly important position in psychiatric theory as a period in which an individual, subject to stress, reaches a crucial point of tension from which either adaptive integration or maladaptive disorganization must eventuate. The significance of crisis, psychotherapeutically, is that at such periods of stress, properly presented interventions can be of maximum efficacy.

The concept of *Developmental Crisis* was originally introduced in relationship to the well-known "Eight Stages of Man" (1). There are indeed many developmental crises throughout human existence, beginning with the process of birth itself. Others include the crucial first year of life, which lays the groundwork for basic security in interpersonal relationships; the acculturation stresses of the second and third years of life, of fundamental importance in connection with the development of inner and outer control mechanisms and relationships to authority symbols; the crisis of the oedipal period, with all of its fateful implications; the separation crises involved in the first school attendance and the first extended departure from home; adolescence; the first employment and heterosexual experiences; marriage, and parenthood.

There is another particularly important crisis period of development, however—the middle years—which, apart from our concern with the gross psychopathologies of menopause, has not received sufficient attention as an inevitable aspect of the aging process in contemporary society.

CAUSATIVE FACTORS

What makes middle age a crisis period? There are four major factors: somatic, cultural, economic, and psychological.

Somatic Factors

As individuals reach the middle years of life, the *somatic* evidences of the aging process can no longer be ignored. There comes a moment in the life of every man and woman when the decreased elasticity of the skin, the accumulating wrinkles, and the coarsening of the features can no longer be ignored or denied by the psychologically healthy person. There is the inevitable fateful day when reading glasses are prescribed for the first time, or when a man, catching sight of the back of his head in a three-way mirror, realizes that the balding person at whom he is looking is no other than himself. For the woman there is the sagging of breasts once proudly firm, the beginning of irregularity of menstruation, and then the finality of its cessation. For both men and women, there are the slackening of muscular activity and the tendency toward increase in weight, with the never-ending subsequent struggle between oral craving and oral frustration. Quite apart from any specific pathologic syndromes, the normal somatic changes that accompany the middle years constitute a series of critical emotional stresses for all people, the significance and impact of which, however, vary in different individuals for reasons that shall presently be discussed.

Cultural Factors

The second important area of stress is the *cultural* one. This is especially relevant in the United States where youth and physical vigor are particularly valued. One might speculate that the high valuation of these patterns in American culture may be a carry-over of our frontier history where such physical attributes were indeed essential for survival. Regardless of its source, however, it is worth noting that this is a peculiarly potent aspect of American cultural life which does not exist in the same degree in older European and Asian cultures, where middle-aged people are still considered attractive and desirable and where the elderly receive considerably more respect and appreciation. Consequently, in the context of

American culture, the beginning loss of youth and vigor is a relatively more severe narcissistic injury.

Still another relevant factor in American cultural life is the great value placed upon personal success, and the widespread tendency to measure this in terms of prestige, wealth, or power. The failure to have achieved such symbols of success by the time middle age has arrived also, as we shall see, constitutes a significant stress in our milieu.

Economic Factors

The middle years of life also carry with them many increased *economic* stresses. There still exists a prejudice against hiring older people, particularly in business, in both the white- and blue-collar areas; indeed, the increasing advent of automation may increase this discrimination rather than decrease it. Moreover, in an age dominated by complex technology, children require more extended support due to their prolonged training needs, and at the same time, the middle-aged person is often faced with the additional heavy economic burden of supporting aging and ailing relatives. It is possible that this latter burden now will be somewhat eased with the advent of Medicare, but the steady increase of their own medical costs may well continue to represent a serious economic threat to many people in the middle years of life. The insidious diminution in purchasing power which the steady progress of inflation has produced in recent decades constitutes an additional source of strain to most people in this age group.

Psychologic Factors

Most important, however, for the middle years, are the *psychologic* stresses, not only in response to the previously mentioned somatic and environmental pressures, but also to specific emotional factors. Separation loss is a key psychological stress that recurs frequently during this period: the loss of one's youthful self-image, the increased frequency of illnesses and deaths among relatives and friends, the loss of children who leave home, and the loss of love in the "tired" marriage where intimacy has been replaced by mutual toleration and sex takes place without passion or tenderness.

There are two additional, and most significantly stressful factors that affect all middle-aged people, although usually unconsciously. The first of these—already touched upon—involves the loss of the fantasy hopes of youth—the hopes of fame, of accomplishment, of wealth, and of romance. One of the fundamental adjustments that most people have to make in the middle years, if these fantasies have not been achieved, is the facing of the hard fact that their fulfillment has become improbable. This involves a profound problem in self-acceptance and in the willingness and ability to make compromises with inexorable realities.

The second factor—perhaps even a more challenging one—is the fact that the somatic changes of middle age carry with them an inescapable *confrontation with the fact of mortality*. The defenses which have worked so well in youth—the illusion of immortality and the denial of one's own ultimate death—can no longer be maintained. The result is a marked increase in what has come to be known as "existential anxiety," the anxiety that is derived from fully facing both the limits of existence and our own ultimate nonexistence.

An interesting fact, however, is that all of these stresses operate differentially in men and women. In the middle years of life, women manifest psychiatric disorders three to four times as frequently as men do. Why is this so? It is certainly not due to a greater physiologic vulnerability to the aging process. If anything, modern American women maintain their youthful appearance at least as well as men do; indeed, the artifices of the cosmetic industry help them to maintain the illusion of youth far better than men. The evidence strongly suggests, rather, that the reasons for this difference in morbidity are both cultural and psychologic.

First, there is much more emphasis in our culture on the importance of beauty and youth in women as compared to men. Second, the cessation of menses is an obvious narcissistic injury as compared to the more insidious, less visible diminution of virility in aging men. Third, the woman's loss of reproductive capacity at menopause is in direct contrast to the preservation of this capacity in men. Finally, the majority of women in our society still form their identities as mothers and wives, within the family, rather than as persons in the outside world. In middle age, however, the functional role of a woman as a mother and a wife assumes less importance, with children becoming less dependent and the husband less attentive. Consequently, many middle-aged women are apt to feel as though they are being discarded and retired to a cultural ash heap, while men are still able to feel relatively needed and involved in the outside world. (Ironically, this functional difference is reversed in the sixties and the seventies when the woman is apt to find herself much more useful and needed, in the grandmother role, than is the man of comparable age!)

FACTORS CONTRIBUTING TO ADJUSTMENT

Despite these cultural variables, the manner in which these normal stresses of middle life are dealt with in any individual man or woman depends upon factors which are highly personal and idiosyncratic. These factors, for both men and women, are: the basic ego-integrative capacity of the individual—the capacity for flexible adaptation in contrast to emotional rigidity; the nature of interpersonal relationships—the character of the marriage and of the relationship to children, other relatives, and friends; the sense of continuing usefulness—and this depends on the extent of the individual's functional relationships, and the degree of self-fulfillment that they afford; and the breadth of interests in the outside world.

Generally speaking, the weaker the ego-adaptive capacity, the more limited the base of interpersonal relationships, the narrower the foundation of the sense of usefulness and of the interest in the outside world, the more critical will be the impact of the middle-year stresses.

RESPONSE PATTERNS

In general, four major patterns of response to the stresses of middle life can be distinguished.* They are not mutually exclusive, and each, of course, is subject to considerable idiosyncratic variations and blendings.

Denial by Escape

Here, we see people trying to avoid facing their inner anxieties by patterns of compulsive activity. This is why so many middle-aged couples fear being alone with themselves or one another, and are

---

* It should be emphasized that these reactions are typical of contemporary American life, and are not universal for all times and all cultures. Obviously, patterns of adaptation and maladaptation are strongly affected by the mores, the outlets, and the technology of the sociocultural milieu (2).

constantly escaping into the wasteland of TV, or through movies, card games, and parties. The formula that dominates their lives is "What are we doing tonight?"

Denial by Over-compensation

This is another common defense, with efforts concentrated on trying to recapture the lost feelings of youth. Not for nothing are these years sometimes called "the dangerous forties!" The woman utilizing this defense is apt to embark on a desperate search for the romance and the love that has gone out of her marriage, while the man seeks to refurbish his tarnishing narcissistic self-image by pursuing a chain of sexual conquests. As might be expected, this is a crisis period for marriages, and the incidence of divorce reaches a high peak.

Decompensation

If these commonly used defenses fail to work, then we may see various forms of decompensation, with anxiety states, depressive reactions, apathetic surrender, or feelings of rage. (A late Irish poet's anguished cry, "Rage, rage against the dying of the light!") These patterns of decompensation make up what are commonly recognized as the psychologic disorders associated with the menopause.

Integration

On the other hand, if the individual is able to meet the critical developmental stresses of the middle years and deal with them successfully, then the outcome is a state of higher integration than he or she has previously achieved—an integration that means an added dimension of emotional maturity; a heightened awareness of self and of others; a lessening of narcissistic self-involvement and an increase in the capacity to cathect service to others; a greater ability to find pleasure in the achievement of our children, our students, and our youth in general; a renewed capacity for productivity and creativity; and, finally, a deeper appreciation of the complexity and the rich bitter-sweetness that characterize our temporary sojourn on this planet of laughter and tears, "For age is opportunity no less than youth itself, though in another dress." (Longfellow)

REFERENCES

1. ERIKSON, E. H., *Childhood and Society*, W. W. Norton & Co., New York, 1950.
2. McLUHAN, M., *Understanding Media*, McGraw Hill, New York, 1964.

5

Principal Findings Based on Thirty Years' Experience in Endocrine Psychiatry

MANFRED BLEULER, M.D.

Director, Psychiatric Clinic, University of Zurich

Endocrinologic psychiatry illuminates that border area between our purely human, spiritual, and emotional existence, and that dark, elementary, biologic, "animal" background in our psychic life. Clearly, therefore, the first law to emerge is that just as we share hormones with animals, hormones can only affect or directly disturb those hidden areas of our human existence which we have in common with animals. To this we must add a second law: All psychic life processes lurking in the background which can be regulated by hormones can also (even experimentally) be regulated through cerebral, functional systems. It follows, therefore, that hormones exert their influence on the psyche, to which they are geared through functional central nervous systems. This fact has been demonstrated satisfactorily by modern brain physiology.

Which are the psychic life processes that may be altered by endocrinologic factors? They can be readily summarized as motor drive (impulse), periodicity, elementary instincts, disposition (mood), and —in the long run—maturation and aging (development).

Like ourselves, animals may be stimulated or apathetic. Endocrine processes are involved in the interaction between internal causes and the processing of stimuli received from the external environment. We know that stimulation occurs primarily when there is an excess of hormones, and especially when hormone levels begin to rise. Apathy

39

is an even more common phenomenon; it usually accompanies hypo-
functions in the endocrine system and long-term endocrine disorders.
Even in the menstrual cycle, which is regulated by hormones, we can
discern a certain psychic cycle, although it is irregular and often
hard to pinpoint. Gross impairment of time-dependent processes will
often accompany many endocrine diseases, for example, a subjective
feeling of intolerable hunger though the stomach is full or a drive
toward mobility at the wrong time. The cycle between movement in
the small, everyday world and in the large world outside is of particular interest. It is becoming more and more evident to animal
psychologists that the animal is subject to internal, instinctual impulses which, during certain phases of life, confine it to a clearly
limited territory while, at other periods, it will break out into the
great, wide world.

Physiologic processes carry only a small part of the responsibility
for the fact that at one time man feels tied to his home, hearth,
and desk—that is, to everyday life—and at another is inspired to
seek the distant, the different, the new, and the great. Generally,
one will tend to attribute these phases to the instinctive drives of
man on the one hand and to resigned wisdom on the other. Nevertheless, psychopathologic experience has taught us that resounding,
deeply biologic factors are also involved. Many patients with endocrine diseases are suddenly at irregular intervals moved by a
powerful impulse to seek distant shores, and to run away from everyday life, no longer feeling at home in the place where they belong.
But more often we will witness the opposite. Patients with endocrine
disease may be almost paralyzed; mundane events are more important to them than adventure.

Among the elementary instincts which can be influenced by endocrine processes and are attuned to these central nervous functions,
hunger, satiety, and sexuality have been studied extensively. We
call some types of instinctual motherliness "monkey love" (blind
partiality); it has been demonstrated that endocrine processes play
a role in coddling and fondling. The often quite obvious dependence
of aggressive behavior on androgen and other hormones is of particular interest. Mood changes are clearly discernible in almost every
untreated patient with endocrine disease—either instability of moods,
especially in hyperfunctional conditions, or (mainly in endocrine
hypofunction) passive, imperturbable behavior.

Hormones play a continuous role in both physical and psychic development. Retardation, maturation, and aging are common phenomena in endocrine diseases. To some extent the interrelations between a disharmonious endocrine and psychic puberty and a disharmonious physical and psychic climacterium have been elucidated, but some areas are still obscure. Particular interest attaches to the connection between endocrine pubertas tarda and imbecility and between premature climacterium and senile psychoses. That these factors are interrelated has been clearly demonstrated, but we still know far too little about them to be able to draw any practical conclusions. Currently, a great deal of discussion focuses on the question of whether sexual behavior in man—as in a few mammals—is directed toward hetero- or homosexual aims during a certain developmental phase by the presence or absence of androgens. We might conceivably interpret some traits in certain female pseudohermaphrodites in this sense, for instance, in women who have been masculinized by anti-abortion hormone therapy.

There are no psychic life processes which are governed solely by endocrine factors, not even drives, cycles, instincts, moods, or development; various external and internal processes of a psychologic and somatic character are integrated in all of these phenomena. It is remarkable, however, that endocrine factors affect various psychic processes differently; the effect exerted on motor drive is very powerful. It is a heavy burden on those affected and the strain on volition makes this influence by no means innocuous. To convince oneself of this one merely has to observe the torture of the agitated hyperthyroid patient, or, conversely, the deterioration into sloth and filth of patients with Sheehan's disease.

On the other hand, the entire personality puts its imprint on the emerging impulse and affects its bent. The effect of hormones on moods is entirely peculiar to the individual; identical hormone changes may affect mood quite differently in various people. Mood is a much more human and less biologic factor than elementary instincts or motor drive as a whole. We are capable of molding our moods much more consciously according to our life experience and can frequently control them. The philistine may be morose at home but the minute a guest enters, he will be gay and entertaining—certainly not from any endocrinologic causes. Nevertheless, the depressions afflicting patients with endocrine diseases permit the conclusion that endocrine factors have some influence on the quality of mood. What is involved is more a returning toward enhanced or reduced ill humor than a definite mood. Cortisone treatment may produce euphoria or depression among other effects.

Most of our insight into the interrelationship between the psyche and endocrine factors has been gleaned from observing pathologic processes, but it is more difficult to gauge and unravel the connections between psychic and endocrine functions in normal persons. However, we do know now that emotions of all kinds affect endocrine functions within a normal range. Varied emotions have been studied extensively in this respect—anxiety in examinations or fear before operations or a parachute jump, to the excitation of soldiers in a surrounded outpost in the jungles of Vietnam. Investigation of the latter (1) has provided a vivid example of how an identical external condition may be subject to different internal processing and different emotional reactions, thus arousing diverse endocrine reverberations. Only minor emotional and endocrine reactions were seen in soldiers who performed an accustomed battle task pooling their forces in a group effort, while signal corps men who only had to wait showed strong emotional and endocrine responses. Emotions have an immediate effect on catecholamine release, then affect adrenocortical function, and finally exert a negative effect on gonadotropin secretion. The thyroid gland is less affected by fluctuations in emotional agitation.

We know that endocrine functions depend on emotions, but very little is known of how endocrine functions affect the internal life of healthy persons. Yet enough is known to form a preliminary, basic concept. We know, for instance, that once an endocrine gland has been eliminated, there will often be a slight personality change even if regular substitution therapy is entirely successful according to physical standards. Not infrequently, such patients will be found to be more uniform and impersonal, with a less clearly defined profile and more meager characteristics than the original personality. In such patients emotions no longer affect endocrine functions; and, because of this, it seems that the reaction of the changed endocrine functions on the psyche are also missing. Emotion evaporates more rapidly and becomes less lasting—in other words, less personal.

We also have a rough concept of the psychologic significance of hormones during periods of major physiologic readjustment. A major factor is that there is no psychosexual maturation without hormonal puberty. Hormonal maturation is an absolute prerequisite for personal maturation, although not the only one. Furthermore, it has become quite clear that hormonal development depends largely on interaction between endocrinologic and emotional maturation. Physical puberty in a person whose life experience is meager carries the risk of faulty development. We are now becoming increasingly aware that not only psychosexuality is subject to endocrine influences, but also mature activity, the will to succeed, and—indirectly—faith in one's own strength and independence. Similar interrelationships can be demonstrated for the climacterium and the puerperium, and we can guess that they probably exist in the menstrual cycle.

In the healthy subject endocrine functions prolong and deepen psychic processes. They lend emphasis to emotional arousal and make it more personal. During the developmental period they aid in directing attitudes toward physiologically predetermined, age-conditioned life tasks, not only toward sexuality and elementary motherliness (and, in turn, away from these), but also toward retreat into a narrower world of active accomplishment, and they help the individual to mature physiologically.

Patients with endocrine diseases are also affected psychically. Although this is partly owing to the torturous experience of physical changes, the immediate hormonal effects on and through the brain are also implicated. Such patients need humane psychotherapeutic care, aid, and attendance. They rarely require special psychiatric therapy, and psychoanalytic treatment in particular is seldom feasible. They need physicians who will devote time to them, be interested in their condition, and advise them in their distress. Above all, they need physicians with whom they can feel safe, and in whose care they find rest and security. The frequency with which these patients do indeed find such physicians is impressive. With this type of patient the ancient art of the physician has not changed; he must treat the patient's physical ailment, must at the same time be close to him, and—in the most comprehensive sense of the term—also be his psychotherapist.

REFERENCE

1. BOURNE, P. G., et al., *Arch. Gen. Psychiat.*, 19:135-140, 1968.

6

Phase-Specific Therapy of Psychic Disturbances: Biologic, Psychotherapeutic and Sociodynamic Aspects

HANS HOFF, M.D.* and
GUSTAV HOFMANN, M.D.

The time of unilateral causal research in psychiatry is now a matter of the past. Investigators everywhere in the world are now attempting to combine biologic aspects with psychopharmacologic criteria and in-depth psychology.

When proponents of psychoanalysis originally ventured forth from Vienna, this new school of thought was viewed as the antithesis by those oriented towards purely organic criteria. At that time, the latter group, and those who held that not only neuroses, but even psychoses, could be treated solely by psychotherapy, were divided into two bitterly opposed camps. This narrow view is now antiquated, and it is hard to imagine that such a one-sided approach could ever again occupy a dominant position.

The rift between these two schools has long been bridged and it can be said with a certain measure of justification that the Viennese Clinic has made some contribution to this rapprochement regarding research into both causation and therapy.

These studies, and the findings they have produced, have repeatedly illustrated that any extreme point of view on the therapy of a sick man is out of place. It is known that the psychotic patient is affected in all areas, in the depth of his personality, as well as in his auto-

---

* Deceased. Formerly, Dean of Medicine, University of Vienna.

nomic nervous system, and sometimes even in the functioning of the brain itself. It is believed that some emphasis should be placed on various forms of therapy, as they relate to the phase of the disease.

The author differentiates between neuroses and psychoses, but believes that in each instance of psychosis, there is a coming to terms between the individual personality and the impending disturbance. Therefore, from a nosologic point of view, we adhere to the concept of a formal disturbance (psychosis) which is not determined by its content. We admit, without hesitation, however, that the life history of the patient is involved in the content around which a psychosis is built up (i.e., in the delusional idea or the object of depressive concepts of fear), and this represents a specific personality reaction.

We also take cognizance of the fact that man, including man suffering from a disease, does not live in isolation, but in a community, and after hospitalization he will again return to the community of the family, the group at his place of work, and the circle of his friends.

Based on these concepts, and viewing the genesis of psychosis as determined by multifaceted factors, a brief survey of the phase-specific therapy conditioned by these multifarious dimensions is offered here, and this can best be done by describing the longitudinal course and the longitudinal therapy of an acute schizophrenic psychosis.

In the author's clinic, acutely psychotic patients are sometimes admitted by compulsory hospitalization ordered by the health officer. Every person reacts to a restriction of his freedom with excitement, which—in the acutely psychotic—may be further excessively elevated due to a psychotic fear. In this situation, the patient will be most distrustful and rejecting towards the physician and nursing personnel. Therefore, it is thought that at this time, psychotherapy can only consist in the offer of a benevolent, rather indifferent, attitude on the part of the physician, reserving the continuity of the therapeutic environment until later. Any attempt to exert a direct influence by means of psychotherapy oriented towards depth psychology would appear to be hopeless as well as uneconomical at this point.

During this phase of psychosis, drug therapy and biological methods must necessarily be the treatments of choice. In the present time, it is fortunate that there are now psychopharmacologic drugs that enable the physician to manage any type of excitement, irrespective of its genesis. Electroshock therapy is only necessary in exceptional circumstances (for instance, in acute catatonia threatening lethal consequences). The rather nonspecific approach to initial therapy, as described here, attenuates excitement, prevents aggression from the patient, and at the same time it also goes far towards suppressing fear in both patient *and* nursing personnel.

By reducing the fear of the "insane," which often even affects physicians, the therapeutic environment of the psychiatric clinic is made more humane. The patient is considered a sick person and treated accordingly.

It is important to emphasize that this type of therapy is quite independent of the individual patient's personality. It is quite immaterial whether the patient comes from a higher or lower socioeconomic level, or what cultural group he belongs to.

Furthermore, using this type of therapy, the physician gains time to arrive at a more precise diagnosis. He can afford to wait with certain additional examinations (involving, for instance, neurophysiologic or psychologic techniques) until the patient's inital excitement has abated.

In the second phase of the treatment, a more precise diagnosis is imperative. In addition to nosologic classification of the syndromes observed, evaluation of psychologic defense mechanisms, which are closely related to the individual personality, now begins to play a more important role. This means that, in addition to nosologic diagnosis, the physician must gain at least preliminary insight into the psychodynamics operative in each instance. Also at this time, all problems which emanate from the sociologic entanglements involved in the disease picture must be evaluated.

During this second phase, treatment of the respective disease will proceed (more or less specifically) with particular attention to the nosologic classification. For this purpose, it is necessary to differentiate between psychoses and behavioral disturbances on the one hand, and within the class of psychoses (between manic-depressive disease and schizophrenia, or psychoses with a physical base) on the other hand; also, a more precise subclassification according to each target syndrome is necessary.

During this second phase, then, the more or less specific therapeutic methods will begin to be used, for instance, antidepressives, electro-

or insulin shock in depressions; or the neuroleptic drugs in schizophrenic patients. At the same time, however, discussions of the conflict situations will be started in the psychologic sphere, depending on the possibility of making contact with the patient and his capability to bear the stress. It is considered to be most important to start psychotherapy during this phase, which may be called the stage of early rehabilitation.

It has long been known that the prognosis of a disease does not depend only on the factors which constitute the disease (this is especially true of schizophrenia), but also pertains to relapses of depression, and to some extent, even neuroses. To a large extent, regression of the disease and the social adaptation of a mental patient will depend on the success of the adjustment between the personality of the individual and his environment. This adjustment may be disturbed to the same extent by a wrong neurotic attitude as by an unfavorable environment, such as the absence of a place to work. In analogy, psychotherapy, or intervention in the social sphere, may influence adaptation decisively. It is clear that during this phase of rehabilitation, the worries and problems of the individual, his unique personality structure, and the environment in which he is placed, will be the sole determinants for suitable therapeutic measures.

We have seen, then, that in the sense of a multi-conditional therapy, during the acute condition the emphasis of treatment was on an entirely nonspecific therapy, but it is also clear that such less-than-specific drug therapy and physiologic therapeutic measures alone do not suffice to assure the mentally-ill patient optimal therapy. The more the classic symptoms of the disease, which are more or less the same for everyone all over the world, recede into the background, the more dominant will be the personal problems and cares of the individual. These demand highly differentiated treatment, depending on each individual personality structure. At this stage, an attempt must be made to achieve a good balance between the individual's personality and his own environment.

It is necessary to appraise the various layers of the personality afflicted by the disease and their capacity to affect the disease process and the therapy properly, and confront this with an adequate phase-specific therapy. Only then will optimal treatment have been provided according to modern insight into the etiopathogenesis of psychic disturbances.

7

Comprehensive Psychiatric Models and the Physiology of Behavior

HAMILTON F. FORD, M.D.

Professor and Chairman, Department of Neurology and Psychiatry, University of Texas, Medical Branch

"Despite the claim of Freud, its creator, that psychoanalysis is based on biological knowledge, his disciples have so heavily emphasized the autonomy of psychological process that two-way bridges between dynamic psychology and physiology have been few" (1).

Psychiatry has never been deficient in conceptual models. In every era the student of psychiatry could choose from a long list of possibilities or exercise his imagination in deriving a new theoretical schema. Wallace's quotation, however, points to an important aspect of theoretical psychiatry—its tendency to produce intellectual enclaves that develop more or less mutually exclusive systems or perspectives. Not infrequently these enclaves receive their initial impetus from theoretical work in other behavioral science disciplines, but once incorporated into the thinking of psychiatry they tend to become stereotypical and to draw for the most part on speculation within the intellectual framework for further elaboration.

Wallace's remarks, made from a position outside psychiatry looking in, point to psychoanalysis as some sort of scientific culprit whose preoccupation with its own psychologic constructs makes a meaningful dialogue with other systems of thought impossible. This may be a valid observation, but before assigning blame, the student of biologic or physiologic psychiatry should objectively reevaluate his own position and that of his colleagues.

The sheer number of past and present models for explaining deviant behavior attests on the one hand to the inadequacy of these concepts and, on the other, to the lack of core reference data for validating or rejecting proposed models. The biologic approach has had its successes: for example, in general paresis, mongolism, phenylketonuria, and temporal lobe tumor. In a broader sense, however, the understanding of more subtle variations on the homeostatic theme has been less successful. Whether a better understanding (that is, a more comprehensive model) of behavior might be obtained through dialogue with other theoretical perspectives remains to be seen. The biologic psychiatrist has not been all that eager to build "two-way bridges."

The current trend in much of psychology, sociology, and anthropology is toward theoretical synthesis, and such rubrics as behavioral science, social psychology, and psychologic anthropology reflect this new thrust. Many investigators in these fields eagerly seek points of theoretical congruence for the sake of the heuristic questions implicit in the congruence. The emphasis is on continued dialogue rather than defense of the traditional limits of explanatory models. Where different levels of integration can be identified, new and innovative synthesis may be possible. The motivation for such an effort is explicit in a passage written by Redfield (2) in 1941:

> "The world of science and scholarship rests on qualities of common understanding that tempt one to look upon it as the beginning of an integration wider than has existed before."

This denial of territoriality in the behavioral sciences must, of necessity, raise important questions for all behavioral scientists including the physiologic psychiatrist. Not the least of these is the degree to which cross-fertilization can contribute to the development of new and more comprehensive models of health and psychologic impairment. Recent developments in research relating to the biology of behavior hint at the biologic psychiatrist's role as a contributor, and his unique position as a biologic theorist who must implement his theory in social settings provides an almost ideal situation for bridge building.

In the early 1950s Heath (3) at Tulane began reporting the results of in-depth electrode placement in human beings. He identified central

nervous system (CNS) areas, the septum in particular, where elec-
trophysiologic abnormalities were associated with psychotic behavior.
Additional work by the Tulane group led to reports of a serum factor,
presumably a protein moiety, isolated from schizophrenic patients.
The appearance of these reports precipitated a sometimes heated
debate at psychiatric meetings and in the literature. Subsequent
work by Gottlieb and his co-workers (4) at the Lafayette Clinic in
Detroit resulted in the identification of a similar factor that, according
to the authors, provides a basis for a tentative separation of disease
entities within the descriptive category of schizophrenia. Similar
work is being reported by Bergen and his associates (5) from the
Worcester Foundation for Experimental Biology, and from European
centers.

Whether the factors described by the various authors reflect an
inheritable physiologic disturbance, an exogenous viral substance, a
physiologic concomitant of experiential ontogeny, or a normal variant
remains controversial. It is not impossible that the answer could be
forthcoming from investigations based on a dialogue with the representatives of other perspectives. The evidence, recently offered by
Heath and Krupp (6), for an autoimmune component in psychosis
only serves to enhance this possibility. The impact of inculturation
on amine metabolism, the effect of interpersonal stimulation on developing CNS cell stations, and the part played by experience in autoimmune mechanisms are all questions requiring models more comprehensive than are possible at a purely physiologic level. At the
same time, however, adequate heuristic models are impossible without
a physiologic perspective.

The relationship of amine metabolism and neurotransmitters to
affective states has recently received a great deal of attention. The
initial impetus for this work was the introduction of effective tranquilizers and antidepressants, but the theoretical formulation of
Schildkraut (7), then at NIMH, in assembling fragmentary data
into a hypothetical model facilitated this interest. Schildkraut has
labeled this model the "catecholamine hypothesis of affective disorders." In brief, he proposes that depression is related to a decrease
in catecholamines at adrenergic receptor sites in the CNS, while
elation is associated with an excess of these agents. The value of his
effort lies not only in its organization of previously uncorrelated
data, but in its primarily being an example for future efforts aimed

at synthesization and conceptualization. Again, these future efforts may be enriched by two-way bridges that serve to link the social, the psychologic, and the biologic.

Sleep physiology has recently provided an unexpected and fruitful area of research. It has long been recognized that sleep disturbance accompanies many psychiatric syndromes and that the nature of the disturbance is in some instances characteristic of the syndrome. However, it was not until 1953, when Aserensky and Kleitman (8) first observed bursts of rapid eye movements during sleep that the pattern of behavioral and physiologic variables could be correlated. Significant advances have been made in clarifying these patterns in "normal" individuals, and a beginning has been made in describing pattern variations among the psychologically disturbed. These findings provide an opportunity for the simultaneous study of mind (the dream itself) and brain (the dream state). The models for such a study have yet to be developed and require the recognition of congruencies in various theoretical areas.

Other research areas where extensive investigation is in progress include electrolyte metabolism, the effects of somatic therapies, and the mind-altering drugs. A great deal of work is under way in relation to the role of steroid metabolism in modifying behavior and the effect of circadian rhythms on affect and cognition.

Many areas of congruence are emerging in the various areas of physiologic research. Neurotransmitters comprise an important element in amine metabolism and are in turn linked with electrolyte metabolism. Metabolic processes reflect circadian undulations, and almost every physiologic aspect of the human organism is modified during the various stages of sleep. It may be expected that much of this data will, in the near future, be incorporated into new biologic models.

If, however, we are to understand people as they really are, even the most sophisticated physiologic model is inadequate. This reality has not passed unnoticed among physiologic investigators. Pribram (9) has noted points of theoretical congruence between his own physiologic research and that of other investigators in the fields of psychology, sociology, and anthropology. His warning to his scientific colleagues is worth reproducing:

> "I urge that the validity of many conceptual systems can be tested by attention to convergences among them and by testing

these convergences. . . . Without such synthesis through cross-disciplinary effort, science is likely to culminate in a Tower of Babel where the many, by referring to the same event, structured in different realms of discourse, fail totally to communicate."

In the quotation from Wallace (1), which initiated this discussion, the onus of narrow vision rests on the psychoanalyst. Without arguing the appropriateness of Wallace's indictment, it is the responsibility of biologic and physiologic psychiatrists not to hurl vindictive retorts while their own facility in constructing two-way bridges remains in doubt.

The physiologic approach to behavior is critical in the development of more comprehensive psychiatric models. The insights provided by a physiologic perspective will, of necessity, be incorporated into such models. Whether, however, biologically oriented psychiatrists will take an active role in comprehensive model building remains an unanswered question. A general sensitivity to areas of congruence and a predilection to explore those areas are prerequisites for an active role in developing the psychiatric models of the future.

REFERENCES

1. WALLACE, A. F. C., *Culture and Personality,* Random House, New York, 1968. P. 3.
2. REDFIELD, R., In *Modern Systems Research for the Behavioral Scientist,* Buckley, W. (Ed.), Aldine Publishing Co., Chicago, 1968. Pp. 59-68.
3. HEATH, R. G., *Psychosom. Med.,* 17:383, 1955.
4. GOTTLIEB, J. S., et al., In *Biological Treatment of Mental Illness,* Rinkel, M. (Ed.), L. C. Page & Co., New York, 1966. Pp. 334-354.
5. BERGEN, J. R., et al., In *Biological Treatment of Mental Illness,* Rinkel, M. (Ed.), L. C. Page & Co., New York, 1966. Pp. 323-333.
6. HEATH, R. G., & KRUPP, I. M., *Arch. Gen. Psychiat.,* 16:1, 1967.
7. SCHILDKRAUT, J., *Int. J. Psychiat.,* 4:203, 1967.
8. ASERENSKY, E., & KLEITMAN, N., *Science,* 118:273, 1953.
9. PRIBRAM, K., In *The Study of Personality,* Norbeck, E., et al. (Eds.), Holt, Rinehart and Winston, Inc., New York, 1968. Pp. 150-160.

8

Treatment Goals in Psychiatry

NORMAN Q. BRILL, M.D.

Professor of Psychiatry
Center for the Health Sciences, School of Medicine
University of California, Los Angeles

The great demand for psychiatric treatment has stimulated the development of short cuts, crisis treatment, increasing reliance on medication, and social manipulation. Havermann (1) has alluded to the many forms of patching, refurbishing, and expanding the human psyche that have begun to flourish as the influence of psychoanalysis has waned. He says that "by careful count of one observer of the psychotherapeutic scene, there are now no fewer than 200 different schools of thought, most of them very new, on how to make Americans less neurotic, more normal, more 'fulfilled' than they have been in the past." The new schools of thought cover a range from the commonsensical to the exotic. At one extreme are those "who believe that mental disturbances are caused by faulty brain chemistry— at the opposite end are those that have no scientific basis at all, such as the mystical tenets of Yoga and Zen Buddhism."

Intensive psychotherapy and psychoanalysis are increasingly being characterized as uneconomical, wasteful, and even ineffective. There seems to be more interest in effecting changes in society than in the person himself. There is great pressure to utilize lesser trained persons not as assistants, but as independent therapists. Simplistic concepts seem to be replacing early experiences, disturbances in psychosexual development, and instinctual expression as keystones in the understanding of psychopathology. According to Havermann (1), "Some of them promise mind expansion, self realization, self fulfillment, bodily awareness, personal growth, and ecstasy." The goals, then, obviously are not the same. Yet there is a tendency to assume

53

that the results of the various types of treatment are equivalent if symptomatic improvement occurs.

It is no longer a surprise to us that what goes on in treatment may be to gratify something in the therapist (countertransference) and that there is often a discrepancy between what the therapist thinks the patient wants and what the patient actually wants.

Dreikurs (2), in discussing Adlerian psychotherapy, emphasizes the fact that it is always goal directed and that the crucial factor influencing the type of cooperation between doctor and patient is the nature of each other's goals. He says: "In other words, therapy will progress when the goals of the patient and the goals of the therapist are in line with each other. Any resistance is due to the fact that the goals do not coincide."

To the extent that psychiatric disorders are purposeful one can, of course, expect resistance on the part of the patient to giving up his symptoms. The psychiatrist who is trying to remove the patient's symptoms and alter his behavior then has a different objective. But there is a healthy part of the patient's ego that is in alliance with his doctor; this makes him seek help to begin with and it is this part to which attention must be paid.

According to Will (3), in treating a patient it is not necessary that one's theories be right in all respects, but it is important that the therapist be aware of his theories and be willing to recognize their limitations. He states, "The therapist will find it useful to formulate concepts relevant to what he is doing professionally; otherwise his work may be disadvantaged by motivations private and unsystematized that operate out of his awareness."

Just as with somatic diseases, the type of illness should determine the treatment. Unfortunately, the nature of a patient's emotional difficulty is not always as clear-cut as are many of the somatic disorders, and it is more often necessary to do an extended work-up (as has to be done with somatic disorders that are not clear-cut) to determine the nature, extent, and causes of the patient's difficulty. The fact that we are dealing with a whole person and not some particular organ makes the problem much more complex. There are other differences too: the treatment of appendicitis or of a fracture is pretty much the same the world over. Not so with psychiatric disorders, the treatment and significance of which vary from culture to culture.

Of greater importance and more immediate concern is the problem of threading one's way through the confusion of conflicting reports regarding the efficacy of one or another drug; of behavioral modification; and of repressive, expressive, reality, nondirective, and milieu therapies. It is generally not known to what extent the patient's understanding has improved, his attitudes have changed, his interpersonal relationships have varied, and his expectations have modulated.

The variety of treatments that different psychiatrists employ for the same type of psychiatric illness suggests the possibility that their decisions are in part based on their own biases and preferences rather than on the particular disorder. Another possibility is that treatments which are considered more or less specific for certain disorders are in fact not specific. For example, Patient "A" is depressed. An antidepressant drug is prescribed and the patient improves. The physician prescribing the drug may be convinced that the drug has a specific action on depression from the psychiatric literature and from the advertisements he reads in the scientific journals. Another example: Patient "B" is depressed. Uncovering psychotherapy is advised and administered with the physician's conviction that there is an underlying cause for the depression which, when revealed and dealt with, will lead to improvement.

In each instance, when improvement does occur, the physician is inclined to attribute it to what he did, that is, giving a certain kind of medicine or a certain kind of psychotherapy. However, when doctors have been observed while treating patients, it seems that what they report they do differs a good deal from what in fact they do do. In administering drugs the powerful effect of the authority and trust with which the therapist is endowed, and the expectancy of help that the patient has in going to him in the first place, play extremely important roles which will be readily acknowledged, but minimized or forgotten when the virtues of the drug are being extolled. In administering the psychotherapy, nondirective as it may be, great significance will be attached to well-timed remarks and interpretations, while frustrating silences, subtle encouragements, and the fact that this particular patient was selected for treatment rather than some other patient, will receive little credit. The aura of the sessions, which are not interrupted except for emergencies, and the sympathetic manner in which all attention is focused on the patient, tend to be forgotten.

The important question is: Are the results of the different treatment methods the same? Also, are there any specific indications for one kind of treatment as opposed to others? In evaluating the results of treatment, different measures are frequently employed, and even when the same measures are used by different investigators, the measures may not be reliable. One cannot rely merely on change in symptoms, since treatment may relieve a patient of a phobia but disrupt a marriage or be complicated later by the development of a peptic ulcer. Or a patient may overcome sexual frigidity but severe hypertension may develop in its place.

Setting a goal of treatment, therefore, implies an awareness of the complications, the symptom substitutions, and the dependence or independence it carries with it. While patients will generally go along with the treatment the physician recommends or undertakes, they will somehow use it to suit their own purposes and do a lot more directing and pursuing of their own secret goals than the psychiatrist suspects. Patients will even have their own secret time-tables for treatment which are difficult to change even when revealed.

In making rounds on a psychiatric ward, I have often asked patients how long they thought they would need to stay in the hospital, and have been struck by the specific notions so many of them have. Some would say a week, some a month, some six months. Some came to the hospital in the first place to escape the burdens and stresses of their homes, some for the rest or respite from responsibilities. Some came because they were frightened, others because the rest of the family could tolerate them no longer. Some came because they were dissatisfied with themselves; some for sympathy, understanding, and protection; and some to try to understand. I don't mean that they told their motivations in so many words; they would come with the symptoms that were necessary to get them admitted. While they are by no means typical, many of the Veterans Administration's best "customers" admit very frankly that any time they want to come back to the hospital, they tell the admitting office that they are afraid they are going to kill themselves.

One phenomenon that has interested me is that patients (and their families) will often report more improvement from treatment than the psychiatrist is willing to allow. Physicians tend to be much more conservative in their estimates of change; they also tend to be more pessimistic than is justified about what will happen to patients who refuse treatment or discontinue.

Ideally, the goal of treatment should be based on understanding of the patient (not just the psychodynamic and unconscious factors that are operating in the patient's illness) and on what the patient wishes from treatment. Every patient with a hernia does not seek surgery. Some patients just want to be happier, most want relief from annoying symptoms, some want to understand themselves better, some recognize a need for increasing their tolerance for frustration and their self-control, and others may wish to change their personalities. Other factors that need to be considered are the nature and severity of the patient's illness; the age of the patient; his intelligence and physical condition; his psychologic-mindedness and cultural background; his life situation; and, unfortunately, such factors as his financial status and the availability of competent and interested help.

Mental and emotional illnesses are inextricably involved with underlying personality disorders, and in establishing goals of treatment for one, it is necessary to consider the other, especially if one is concerned with long-term as well as short-term results. Because of the tendency to place a higher value on psychotherapy that is designed to help a patient understand his emotional disorder rather than a supportive or repressive therapy that is concerned with symptomatic relief, uncovering or insight-producing psychotherapy may be employed when it is in fact not indicated or is even harmful. On the other hand, purely supportive or repressive techniques are utilized for limited goals when more far-reaching goals would be in the patient's best interest. At times the initial utilization of one particular form of treatment may seriously interfere with the ability to use another later when it becomes clearly indicated.

Automatic and repeated use of shock treatment for patients with neurotic depressions at times results in such passivity and dependence that psychotherapy becomes impossible. The continued use of drugs to relieve anxiety too often these days results in a serious habituation that is often impossible to relieve. On the other hand, there are patients whose fragile egos have been overwhelmed by psychoanalytic approaches that resulted in a chaotic or psychotic thinking disorder and rejection of any kind of somatic approach.

There is much we need to learn about indications for the various types of treatment—an attitude that varies considerably from the often repeated advice that "you've got to believe in one method to be an effective therapist." This is painfully remindful of the witch doctor. Therapists are too often guilty of applying preconceived ideas of psychodynamic causality to patients before understanding the unique background of the individual patients.

In recent years we have seen a turning of attention to the elements in society and the patient's culture that contribute to mental ill health (such as poverty, discrimination, and exploitation). This new approach, called social psychiatry, really got its start in the military services where the quality of leadership, esprit de corps, proper training, fair rewards and punishments, promise of relief from stress, and the buddy system of replacement were recognized as crucial in maintaining individual and group effectiveness. Social psychiatry implies paying attention not only to the elements in society that contribute to a patient's illness, but also to those elements that involve the patient's responsibility to society as exemplified in the military "society."

I expect civilian psychiatry will sooner or later follow the military in the second element of social psychiatry, that is, in shifting the focus from the individual's needs to the needs of society. The individual's effectiveness in fulfilling his responsibility to the needs of the society will then become the goal of treatment—not his happiness nor even his safety especially—as we move more and more to a strong powerful centralized government and as the clear distinctions between states of war and peace become less and less discernible.

REFERENCES

1. HAVERMANN, E., *Reflection*, 5:1-19, 1970.
2. DREIKURS, R., *J. Soc. Issues*, 4:39-54, 1948.
3. WILL, O. A., "Schizophrenia Versus Psychological Treatment." In *Comprehensive Textbook of Psychiatry*, Freedman and Kaplan (Eds.), Williams and Wilkins, Baltimore, 1967.

9

Obnoxiousness in Psychiatric Patients and Others

PETER A. MARTIN, M.D.

Clinical Professor of Psychiatry,
Wayne State University School of Medicine
and the University of Michigan Medical School

The Psychiatric Forum offers its contributors an opportunity to speak freely on any subject. We are welcome to express personal opinions and convictions free from such encumbrances as lengthy references, which is fortunate for this paper. I can find no references to the subject of obnoxiousness in the psychiatric or psychoanalytic literature. Also, the Forum offers the opportunity to present subjects in early stages of consideration. Stimulating additive responses from the readers contribute to the development of the topic. It is this freedom which allows me to write on the quality of obnoxiousness in psychiatric patients and in non-patients. I have but recently been forced to become aware of its frequency in patients through supervision of psychiatry residents' work at the University of Michigan and Wayne State University. In retrospect, it was like discovering the obvious. A series of patients were presented in whom obnoxiousness was an outstanding complaint of family, ward personnel, and therapists. The lateness of my recognition is surprising since the quality of obnoxiousness is commonly seen in psychiatric patients and particularly among those who are hospitalized. Some of the patients presented would not have been hospitalized and some would have been discharged earlier had the level of their obnoxiousness been lower. The word obnoxious will not be found in any diagnostic manual, but once my curiosity and interest were aroused, the subject continued to be brought to my attention from surprisingly diverse sources. For example, the story of Phillipe Pinel unshackling the inmates at Salpêtrière uncovered an interesting facet: many of the people who were freed from their chains and released were not mentally ill. They were public nuisances, individuals who were obnoxious to the authorities and conveniently removed from the streets by being placed with mentally ill patients who themselves had become obnoxious to their families and society.

Current newspaper reports from Russia indicate that individuals who are critical of the government are declared mentally ill and hospitalized for years. In many communities in the United States laws have been in effect for many years that make it a punishable offense to be "undesirable, objectionable, or generally obnoxious." That these laws are enforced selectively has but recently led to controversy and to a Supreme Court decision that struck down a Cincinnati ordinance making it a misdemeanor for "three or more persons to assemble on any of the sidewalks and there conduct themselves in a manner annoying to persons passing by." The Court declared the ordinance unconstitutionally vague because of individuals could not know in advance when they might be committing a crime.

This pattern continues to be seen to this day. There are psychotic patients who are treated without hospitalization. Hospitalization takes place for many reasons—one of them being to get an "obnoxious" person out of the family. The most striking clinical example of this phenomenon is the manic-depressive personality. During the depression the patient is sad, experiences inner pain, is uninterested in caring for himself, and is to a degree a burden on the family. The patient may even ask to go into a hospital but the family refuses, stating that the patient is no big burden. The depressed keep to themselves in their low periods and cause little irritation. Gradually, as the patient's depressed mood lifts, the family is delighted as the patient is now active, helpful, and a pleasure to be with. In a typical case, the patient, feeling good, cleaned the house, went shopping for new clothes, had her hair done, and prepared dinner for the family. But she continued on into hyperactivity in which she became loud, threatening, seductive, combative, angry, critical, and insomniac. The patient, expressing her pleasure with life, felt no need for treatment. The family stated that she was now obnoxious and wanted her committed. This is a common picture in manic-depressive histories.

Obnoxiousness is one of the characteristics of the manic state. Other diagnostic categories also include this characteristic.

One patient, diagnosed as borderline character, was hospitalized because of verbal and physical battles with his wife and remained hospitalized because of similar battles with attendants and nurses. He would repeatedly criticize others for not doing what he thought they should do for him. It was clear that his reality testing was defective. His irritating approach did not cause others to give him the attention and love which he demanded. Not only is reality testing defective in obnoxiousness but there is also a lack of capacity for empathy. What is missing is an awareness of the other person's needs, problems, and capacities to respond. Obnoxiousness derives from the individual's narcissistic preoccupation with himself and his own needs as being the only fact of social relevance.

Another patient could not readily be placed into any official diagnostic nomenclature. We "diagnosed" him as character disorder-obnoxious character. He had been expelled from professional school not because of scholastic inadequacy but because he would in effect tell his professors that they did not know what they were talking about. He could not understand why they took offense. When he was working, he walked into the boss' office, sat at his desk, and used the telephone for a personal call. When the boss walked into the office and stood there watching him, the patient continued talking for minutes and later could not understand why his boss was upset. His girlfriend found him obnoxious, moved out of town, and became engaged to another man. He was very upset. He was sure she loved him, did not mean the horrible things she had said about him, and that she was waiting for him to come and rescue her.

Paranoid personalities are another category of patients in whom the quality of obnoxiousness intrudes upon interpersonal relationships. Their suspiciousness, distrust, denial of reality, attributing of hostile qualities to the other person, and inability to comprehend evidence to the contrary contribute to their being experienced as obnoxious individuals.

Some sociopaths are an interesting paradox in terms of obnoxiousness. At times they are the opposite of obnoxious. They can be so charming and personable that they have little difficulty in using and abusing other people. They have an ability to locate the weaknesses in the other person's reality testing and subtly to distort reality. It may be only after long suffering that the victim sees through the deceptions and in self defense becomes outraged and indignant. Many therapists have found themselves in such predicaments. When the erstwhile victim attempts to reestablish the reality which he holds valuable, strong feelings of negativism arise and the sociopath is experienced as obnoxious.

Physicians have a common term for a type of patient whom they find obnoxious. They call them "crocks" and attempt to get rid of them by referral to psychiatrists. These so-called crocks are hypochondriacal patients. Repeated examinations disclose no organic reasons for the chronic complaints of the patient, who is not swayed in his needed conviction that he has a physical ailment. This attack and distortion of the physician's reality evokes strong countertransference reactions in the physician, causing him to abdicate his position as a physician and to rid himself of this irritating hypochondriacal distorter of reality.

The reader can readily visualize or has experienced the therapeutic atmosphere present with such patients. They pay little attention to interpretations and negate disdainfully any interpretation which is not supportive of their wishes. In therapists, feeling frustrated and thwarted, negative countertransferences may develop. In a therapeutic relationship the psychiatrist stands for reality. The reality as he sees it is the foundation from which his interpretations to the patient proceed. When, for example, a psychiatrist stated reality as he clearly saw it ("you cannot expect every girl to go to bed with you on the first date; she may have feelings and needs of her own which are contrary to your wishes"), he expected the patient to recognize and accept the validity of this statement of the obvious. When, instead, the patient laughed condescendingly and with great assurance refuted the statement, the patient was experienced as obnoxious, enraging, or psychotic.

Marion Milner's account of a psychoanalytic treatment, *The Hands of the Living God* (1), and Peter Giovacchini's review (2) of her book, help us to understand such periods of disturbed personal relations between patient and therapist. Mrs. Milner and her patient, Susan, often experienced peace and contentment when the dominant transference theme was symbiotic fusion. Such conditions are often nonthreatening and do not disrupt the course of treatment. In contrast, Mrs. Milner describes her discomfort when Susan behaved in an organized manner. When Susan's paranoia effectively made use of secondary process elements, the therapist experienced her wish to drop the treatment. Dr. Giovacchini describes his own reacting with irritation to one of his patient's well developed paranoid system, a reaction to the rational arguments the patient presented to support his delusional system. The paranoid superstructure clothes psychotic mechanisms in secondary process elements. Giovacchini states, "The closeness of such a superstructure to external reality, and especially a reality the patient senses the therapist may be especially interested in, makes the maintenance of the analytic setting difficult as it provokes disruptive countertransference reactions."

The greater the obnoxiousness, the more certain there is to be a narcissistic personality structure. The main characteristics of this structure are grandiosity, defect in superego formation, extreme self-centeredness, and lack of empathy for others in spite of eagerness to obtain admiration and approval from them (3). This maintenance of the early narcissistic orientation of the early months of infancy accounts for the defective ego functioning in reality testing as noted throughout the above paragraphs. The obnoxious quality emerges whenever the individual attempts to impose the reality which he values upon the other individual. Of course, he (note the irritable paranoid) experiences the other individual, who does not accept his version of reality, as obnoxious.

In interpersonal relationships people tend to prefer a bit of uncertainty in others. A degree of not being sure, of being anxious, tends to evoke a positive response. In contrast, when someone is absolutely sure of and pleased with himself, and takes other people too lightly, he is often disliked and experienced as obnoxious by the other person.

This material raises the question—why, in contrast, the oft-used expression in psychiatry, the lovable schizophrenic? Certainly the schizophrenic has a serious defect in reality testing. Why then "lovable" instead of the expected term "obnoxious"? Obviously the schizophrenic has a conflict between his ego and reality; but those schizophrenics to whom the term "lovable" is applied have withdrawn into their own world and are not trying to impose it upon others. They wish to be left alone. In contrast, the obnoxious individuals—whether manic, paranoid, phobic, obsessive-compulsive, or hysterical—tend to be bullies, exploiters, and manipulators of other people. When the "lovable" schizophrenic is shut out from the other person's responses, he goes away. When the obnoxious individual is shut out, he tries to break the door down and impose his reality upon the other person. For example, the patient referred to above could not understand why girls would not go to bed with him on the first date. He badgered them until he became obnoxious to them. Obnoxious individuals try to convert others to their own reality. I have seen a case of *folie à deux* in which the psychotic man was obnoxious to his wife. To avoid separating from him or murdering him, she accepted his psychosis. Here we see an individual who is successful in making a convert of another person to his psychotic reality. Once this was accomplished, they both became obnoxious to their families and were both hospitalized.

If my interest in this quality of obnoxiousness were merely to express what has been written above, it might not have been worth presenting in this Forum. There is, however, a broader aspect, that of obnoxiousness in nonpsychiatric patients (the "others" of my title), which has a social significance pertinent to the current American scene of protesters and revolutionaries. Revolutionaries often have the quality of obnoxiousness, John Adams being an outstanding example. As shown in the recent hit Broadway musical *1776*, without Adams' persistent, demanding, urging, manipulating, maneuvering, and exploitation of others, the Declaration of Independence would neither have been written nor signed. America might have remained a colony under British domination. Yet even his own colleagues who were on his side, such as John Hancock and Benjamin Franklin, could not stand him and found him obnoxious. His principles and vision were proven by history to be correct. His contention that allowing slavery to continue was contrary to the spirit of the Declaration of Independence was patently so. But his manner of trying to force it down the throat of the South was obnoxious to all. He failed. Yet, had he succeeded, the Civil War might have been avoided and the present day dilemma of black-white confrontations avoided. The point that history seems to make is that one should not be distracted by the quality of obnoxiousness from the possible validity of the ideas being verbalized. Certainly this is true for psychiatrists listening to the content of their patients' presentations. The critical observations about the wife of the patient who was hospitalized because of his fighting with her turned out in time to be an accurate evaluation. The critical comments (which kept him hospitalized) about the attitudes of the nurses, attendants, and inadequate ward supervision were known to be valid and a cause for continuous training of ward personnel. His personal problem was that he was incapable of walking away from his wife or from the ward personnel. He needed to break their doors down and change them. But there was validity to his ideas.

In all societies throughout history, statements or positions taken by individuals considered obnoxious were routinely ignored. When the same position was later taken by a member of the elite, it was treated with respect. The point of this presentation is that we can learn important things from individuals who may be experienced as obnoxious. Even the wildest paranoid delusion has a kernel of truth for which we search as a starting point in our working relationship with the patient; so must we do with any so-called "obnoxious" individual. Even though we may consider him lacking in good taste, manners, loyalty, patriotism, appreciation, gratitude, or humility, our capacity for empathy can separate the various parts and rescue the baby from the dirty water. In addition, some of the most revolutionary ideas, such as those of John Adams, later become accepted as "of course" or "old hat" as newer ideas evolve.

Psychiatrists are experts in selling important ideas in a nonobnoxious manner. They should also be experts in accepting important ideas even if presented in an obnoxious manner. The touchstone for this capacity of separating content from manner of presentation is the ingredient which is notably lacking in the "obnoxious" person. It is the ingredient for which the psychiatrist is especially noted— the capacity for empathy. The capacity to understand what another person is feeling and to transmit this understanding to the other person is the antidote for obnoxiousness in ourselves.

REFERENCES

1. Milner, M., *The Hands of the Living God,* International Universities Press, New York, 1969.
2. Giovacchini, P., *Psychiat. Soc. Sci. Rev.,* 5: 22-28, May 26, 1971.
3. Kernberg, O. F., *J. Amer. Psychoanal. Assoc.,* 18: 51-85, 1970.

Section II
SOCIAL PSYCHIATRY

10

Man's Work and What It Means

FRANCIS J. BRACELAND, M.D.

Senior Consultant, Institute of Living (Hartford, Conn.)
Editor, American Journal of Psychiatry

Among the many faults which today's young folks find with their parents' generation is its propensity to look upon work and economic security as being of paramount importance. True enough, the young are enabled to protest because they are being supported and educated by the fruits of parental labors, but that fact is overlooked in the enthusiasm of their "activism." At another end of the scale altruists are concerned as they note the nation's rising unemployment rate, for they know that this of necessity must add to the nation's economic and cultural woes and to the distress of thousands of families.

These factors, plus the large number of older men who are yearly being forced into retirement, attract the attention of psychiatrists to the emotional accompaniments of man's work and also to the lack of it. Fortunately physicians are rarely unemployed and rarely retire completely, so they do not experience these problems firsthand. The loss of a job, especially for a man with a family, is often an ego-shattering blow, and though we as physicians can do nothing about the ebb and flow of the nation's labor market rate, we can be of assistance to individuals and families if we are able to take into consideration of their symptoms the emotional problems of people at work and of people out of work.

Despite voluminous writings concerning the various aspects of man's work, produced through the ages, it is strange that no one has been able to define work satisfactorily. Everyone admits that it is a purposeful activity expected of adult males in our culture, and

69

all agree that it exerts a compelling influence on his personal, inter-personal, and social behavior and relationships; but that is where agreement usually seems to end.

Other reactions are paradoxical. What for one man is work, for another is play, and vice versa. Depending upon the person, the age period, and the cultural beliefs, it has been regarded as either a bless-ing or a curse, as joy or drudgery, as saintly or sinful.

To the Greeks and the Romans work was a burden; the ancient Hebrews considered it drudgery; and the early Christians thought of it as punishment that had to be endured. Man worked because he and his family were hungry. "In the sweat of thy brow shalt thou eat bread." But through the centuries the goals of work expanded and slowly began to rise above the satisfaction of purely physiologic needs. The Calvinists taught that it was God's will that man should work and they considered idleness a sin. They did not discourage an honest search for wealth as a by-product as long as profits were shared with others or used for the general welfare rather than for the pur-suit of worldly pleasures. This attitude toward work and money was perhaps the first indication of the present-day economic trend of capitalism, which is the *bête noire* of activist groups of all shades and sizes.

Various writers have extolled work and idleness. Carlyle believed that endless significance lay in work; he spoke of man perfecting himself by working. Undoubtedly work does give a man a feeling of identity that nothing else does. It serves to regulate his activities, enforce self-discipline, and enhance his self-esteem. Much to the dis-tress of their wives, a great majority of men feel that it is by their work that they validate themselves.

However, not all writers have agreed with Carlyle. Robert Louis Stevenson felt that work dwarfed the soul, yet he himself was a prodigious worker. Besides, extremes are not the rule—a middle course is possible between devoting one's life completely to labor and coasting along in idleness—and it is this middle course that most of us pursue.

It seems axiomatic, therefore, that incontrovertible statements can-not be made about the importance of work or of leisure in anyone's life or about the proportion of each that is necessary to happiness and emotional well-being. Labor has its rewards and so has leisure, and both have their dangers. We can interpret their respective merits only in the light of personal inclinations and emotional attitudes, individual circumstances, and the trend of the times in which we live.

We can add to the reasons why psychiatrists should be interested in work and unemployment:

1. Man does not become ill or exhibit this in a vacuum; he becomes ill in his daily surroundings, and since he spends half of his waking hours at work, it becomes the stage upon which a large portion of the drama of his life is played.

2. It has been demonstrated that by far the greatest proportion of dismissals in industry results from emotional and personality problems rather than from technical inepititude. It is also estimated that the greatest cause of absenteeism, after the common cold, is some form of temporary emotional upset, even though it manifests itself in physical symptoms.

3. Prevailing unrest and personality problems can render working conditions untenable; hence offices, schools, and various institutions have been known to have serious disruptions owing to personality clashes among employees.

4. The conditions under which individuals work are changing rapidly in the culture; some individuals have difficulty in adapting to rapid change and are destined to fall by the wayside.

An outstanding psychiatrist (1) interested in social issues once gave an excellent description of what work and the loss of it means to an individual:

> In our civilization work is what man lives by. . . . We work to earn the necessities of life, to secure its comforts, to provide as befits a man for our families. It helps still the feelings of inferiority that unconsciously beset us; it gains us parity with our fellows and the acceptance of the community. It dignifies our daily life, no matter how humble. In it we may expend our aggressive impulses and ward off the profound feelings of insecurity and helplessness. With work man earns more than a stipend; he gains the right to be master in his home.

For the unemployed man all of this has changed and his most pressing need is to maintain his position in the home and family. If his unemployment is protracted, "life deteriorates into a sodden repetition of job-seeking and lounging about the house. He no longer meets his fellows on the job, and whatever limited camaraderie was his no longer exists" (1). It is probable that in this poignant description of the emotional reactions of the unemployed man is to be found a much better definition of the meaning of work than any we might be able to concoct here. We have to keep in mind also that at home man is seen in a different light than he is at work. He rarely goes to work when drunk or in one of his worst moods. Therefore, work becomes a fundamental resource, a face to show to society, something to hold on to as long as possible.

In many ways, work is the expression of the human being. It means more to him than the financial security and ability to buy merchandise that he finds attractive; and for some people, especially those in appropriate jobs, work is pleasurable. Also work can satisfy, at least in part, certain basic emotional needs. One of these needs is to achieve a sense of mastery at work; the exercise of a skill is an exercise in self-expression. Work is also the purveyor of prestige and other intangibles such as recognition for a task well done or the satisfaction of discharging responsibilities with care. Further, a job has meaning when it provides the satisfaction of fellowship and status in a group. A sense of belonging, of being a part of a group struggling toward a common goal, helps a man identify with what he is doing; he can visualize the work in a larger context and understand the ultimate purpose of his labors. He feels needed when he knows that he is contributing to the completion of a product that has social usefulness. When work fulfills most of these needs, a man can be content in his job and produce at his highest level.

But all too often work fails to provide the emotional gratification that men need. This is one of the disadvantages of many modern industrial settings—work becomes less personal, more mechanized, and the emotional aspects are neglected or forgotten. Everyone cannot get the kind of work he wants when and where he wants it, and important human needs have to be suppressed in favor of economic considerations. Some jobs, for instance, fail to offer an adequate outlet for man's instinctive energy, particularly his aggressive energy. No employer can commit himself to provide meaning and stimulation free of stress or anxiety in a work situation. Many tasks, in their unending sameness, by their very nature, wreck a man's creativity. Daily monotony is not a tasty dish for people. Yet, we all know how relative and subjective the feeling of monotony can be. Some days even an extremely varied professional job may seem unbearably pedestrian; a task done one day with enthusiasm can scarcely be tolerated the next. And what may be monotonous and completely undemanding for one person may be stressful and threatening for another.

Threatening pressures imposed by the job, and its failure to provide adequate emotional outlets, result in a state of tension in the worker. There is no doubt that undue emotional tensions are the insidious enemy and at times even the eventual destroyer of the well-being of industrial employees. Industrial psychology, which has demonstrated and illuminated some of the problems of industrial relations, has also shown that many hazards of industrial activity reside neither in machines nor in a toxic environment, but in a toxic psychology in those who operate the machines. It becomes apparent, therefore, that a combination of unsatisfactory working conditions or personal circumstances may upset the worker, lessen his performance, and cause him to lose zest for his job. The problems that ensue are not easy to deal with and, in fact, may be hard to recognize. But it is clear that they can assume tremendous proportions if unchecked. For example, on the present industrial scene difficulties in interpersonal relationships and group morale have increased, absenteeism is a major problem, and alcoholism and personality disorders burgeon. All of these are of emotional origin and take their toll on worker and management alike.

Unfortunately, the psychiatrist, unless he is an industrial physician, can only help with these problems *post facto* for he is consulted only after the emotional problems have reached serious proportions. He can be of help with the retirement problem, however, especially in these days of community psychiatry, by teaching always and everywhere the importance for most men to retire *to* something, rather than to be precipitated into a deadening idleness. Few men are content to do nothing. During their working lives they have looked forward to retirement and its supposed joys, but when the time arrives, the newfound liberty soon begins to pall.

Preparation for retirement should begin in the fifties, yet men are prone to put off considering it, reasoning no doubt that it "will not happen to me," or "they can't get along without me," the latter being a long-standing, widespread delusion. Some forward-looking industrial and business firms are offering "retirement classes" to prospective retireees in an effort to "soften the blow."

It is the man who loses his job and either fails or is delayed in finding another who is in most need of emotional assistance, for the shattering of his ego and self-image has repercussions upon his family. His self-esteem and self-image suffer as he compares himself invidiously with his friends and neighbors. The pathetic trudging about to answer advertisements or apply to agencies, the expectant look of family members as he returns daily to report no progress in finding a job, the bills piling up, the payments due, and even the usual social events add to his feeling of being "out of it," or even useless. Depression is inevitable in many of these individuals; in some it appears early. Undoubtedly the laconic statistics in the daily press noting that the unemployment rate is now up to five percent of the labor force cover a multitude of individual tragedies. The psychiatrist can do little to prevent unemployment; he can keep in mind, however, that loss of work is not only a financial disaster but often also a personal one, and his technical skills may be called for to help depressed individuals and family members in his community practice.

What can be done about the increased leisure time which labor-saving methods and labor laws have brought with them? Nearly 100 years ago the Preamble of the Constitution of the Knights of Labor, dated January 1, 1878, called for "the reduction of the hours of labor to eight per day, so that the laborers may have more time for social enjoyment and intellectual improvement, and be enabled to reap the advantages conferred by the labor-saving machinery which their brains have created." Today, almost a century later, we have more labor-saving machinery than the authors of that document ever dreamed of, and the eight-hour day has long been in effect in most places of business; now, even that has been cut down to 35 hours per week. Vacations are longer and more frequent and, in general, people have more time on their hands than ever before. But do they really reap the benefit of all of this?

This additional time, regrettably, can be used destructively— which is exactly what we must guard against. Young people, in particular, seem likely to get into trouble when time hangs heavily on their hands. Much of the social rebellion and unrest that is so worrisome today arises from the unhealthy use of excess energies not expended during a work day that is often not well motivated and which grows ever shorter. There is always a strong possibility, unfortunately, that some will express themselves through antisocial behavior when they lack constructive outlets for their aggressive energies. This is evidenced in the unrest and riots in the "inner cities."

Many writers have reflected on the negative quality of idleness. Boileau spoke of the terrible burden of having nothing to do and Socrates commented that he is not only idle who does nothing, but he is idle who might be better employed. Before we move on to the positive aspects of leisure, however, it is well to remember that not all time away from one's occupation is leisure time. Crothers has said, "I cannot include under the pleasant name of 'leisure' those activities that are carried on systematically after business hours. Very soon they become things that *must* be done." Admittedly, we are under some compulsion to attend to routine chores during time away from the scene of work. Some of these routines prepare us for the work day; others must be performed to keep our belongings in order, maintain health, carry on a family life, and discharge community and social functions. By way of definition, leisure stresses not freedom from activity, but the freedom to determine one's activities; it implies freedom from compulsion or from routine or continuous work. Leisure does not replace work; both work and leisure are needed for a full life.

According to John Mason Brown, most people spend most of their days doing what they do not want to do in order to earn the right, at times, to do what they may desire. But just what do people desire to do with the hours away from their regular occupations? Leisure cannot be regimented and the type that is good for one person may be anathema to another.

Thus, the emotional reactions of the man at work, out of work, and at leisure are basically the reactions of the man himself as a person. It is the alert family physician who is able to discern the background of the trouble if he is so minded, and of course it is the industrial physician who sooner than any other person in the plant will learn of incipient emotional problems in the personnel. Felton's (2) astute summary of the situation is worth repeating here:

The manifestation of a malfunction in group behavior usually is seen more readily in a symptom presented to the physician than in a year's curve of absenteeism or turnover. It is this variety of clinical events—the tension back pain, the irritability, the recurrent headache, the persistent dermatitis, the urinary frequency, the need for darkened lenses—that demands interrogation of their cause. Most often this will be a cause deeply buried in the morass of historical emotional data.

While work with the unemployed, their families, or with retirees does not hold the excitement that the dynamic search for the causes of neurosis offers, it is nevertheless a part of the physician's function and one which apparently will present itself with increasing frequency in the near future. Gardner holds that self-renewal is one of the most important secrets a society can learn—a secret that will unlock new resources of vitality throughout society. Perhaps the psychiatrist might have a part in that renewal and in the search for that secret in individuals whose difficulties in and out of work have sorely tried them and more often than not in some manner depressed them. In doing so he will become an important agent in helping with a pressing community project.

REFERENCES

1. GINSBURG, S. W., *A Psychiatrist's Views on Social Issues,* Columbia University Press, New York, 1963.
2. FELTON, J. S., *Bull. N. Y. Acad. Med.,* 39: March, 1963.

11

Social Dissonance

RAYMOND W. WAGGONER, M.D., Sc.D.

Professor, Department of Psychiatry
University of Michigan Medical School

Our society today is threatened with a serious breakdown in morale which is present through all levels. Perhaps the greatest degree of disruption occurs through lack of opportunity and sense of accomplishment in the minority groups. Whatever the source of this difficulty, it most assuredly is not the obvious one, since these obvious conditions have existed for generations. One particularly significant factor is the great discrepancy between socially determined values and the reality function of those values. Although the hippies, Yippies, and college radicals are, according to the news media, among those responsible for the prevailing dissonance, it is apparent that this is only a superficial interpretation. That each era has seen a rebellion of sorts emphasizes that the present social problems have a deeper significance. Thus, what we see now must be considered an immediate problem with much more serious and stubborn problems in the background. Ingle (1) states:

> I do not accept the explanation that the behavior of student and non-student activists is based solely on idealism. There is too much non-think crowd, mob, and frustration behavior, too much public exhibition of infantile anal and genital fixations, too many destructive actions and other absurdities. Social change usually can be described in terms of the aggressive minority vs. the passive majority. The majority may not be entirely passive, but restive and permissive. Society should afford the aggressive minority means of rational display but should not permit monopoly by default. This will not satisfy the revolutionist who seeks to destroy the establishment rather than promote social evolution.

But, hopefully, it may avoid malignant outcomes by offering concerned followers of those who lust for power, expanded opportunities for rational communication and debate.

The title of a 1969 conference in which I took part—"Freedom and Rebellion: Whither the Establishment"—seemed to me not only very appropriate but also very audacious in view of the repeated evidence of reaction against the status quo and the obvious dissension which is occurring in our culture at the present time. Unfortunately, the young and militant tend to romanticize the off-beat and the aggressive which, in turn, emphasizes and exaggerates aggressive behavior as a kind of feedback mechanism. Some of what we see is most onerous to those in authority and a stimulant to the rebellious and the militant. It is also a source of concern and dismay to those of us who are older and who presumably represent the "establishment." Much that is being written and said sharpens our dismay. On the other hand, this is in some measure assuaged by the hope and even the expectation that much of the so-called rebellion contains within it the seeds of a better and healthier society.

The rebellion of the young against those in control appears to be worldwide. Revolution or rebellion does seem to have a kind of biologic rhythm. Intolerance can involve many factors besides race; thus, behavior which does not fit into our pattern of values can lead to intolerance. According to Spiegel (2), there have been at least seven cycles of serious civil disorder in our own country since the Stamp Act Riot in 1765. In 1786 there was Shays' successful rebellion of the poor farmers against unjust tax laws; there was the violence of the Protestants against the Irish Catholics in the mid-nineteenth century. The violent Civil War Draft Riots of 1863 resulted from the outrage of poor people who did not have the necessary $300 to buy themselves out of the Civil War draft; at the same time, vicious attacks on Negroes occurred because they were held responsible for starting the War. The West Coast anti-Chinese riots occurred in the 1870s when the "poor whites" of California, angry with the economic competition of the Chinese people and tainted with white racism, led a riot in Los Angeles, killing 23. Similar riots occurred a few years later in San Francisco and Denver. There were the Labor Riots, beginning in 1870 and recurring until the passage of the National Labor Relations legislation in the 1940s. Horrendous anti-

Negro riots occurred before and after World War I in which a vicious outbreak of white racism led to uncontrolled aggression, including clubbing, shooting, and lynching of Negroes.

Since 1964, of course, there have been numerous instances of black people using violent methods in attempts to achieve what they believe is a more equitable status in our society or to erode the power structure. Similarly, the young and militant are rebelling in the universities to achieve comparable ends; that is, to have more to say about their own destinies. This unhappy cyclical history of violence in our country seems to be correlated with chronic social conflict and may be symptomatic of a basic flaw in its social structure, demonstrated by the incompatibility between our democratic ideals and our authoritarian practices.

Psychiatrists should play a role as the "living link" in the generation gap and should be a vital catalyst in the interrelationship of the generations. This they can do if they keep themselves alert to social change and equipped with psychologic and social means to cope with the task. Spiegel (2) states:

> Violence as the maximum arousal of aggression for destructive purposes, including the killing of one's own species, is, by the same token, an innate behavior potentially capable of being aroused in all men. But the internal, biologic conditions necessary for arousal are ordinarily under the control of external, environmental contingencies. If this view is correct, then what is sorely needed is research directed at investigating the feedback relations between the mechanisms of biologic arousal, particularly in childhood, and the environmental controls, both instigating and inhibiting over-aggressive behavior.

It is our responsibility to initiate and develop research, and to try constantly to bring democratic ideals in line with social practice.

It should be of particular concern to us that once a pattern of hostility and aggression is firmly established, it tends to continue and perhaps even to increase whether or not the original stimulus is appropriate or continuing. A noted example of this type of development is the Mafia of Italy which developed from a legitimate rebellion of the peasants against the Baron overlords, but continued to develop and function even though the basic premise no longer existed. When the Mafia chieftains were driven out of Italy, they immigrated to the United States and have continued to develop aggressive criminal behavior of this sort which, once established, tends to feed on itself and to spread rather than to be self-limited. The wide variety of ethnic and geographic groups immigrating to this country has no doubt contributed to our enormously rapid and remarkable techno- logic developments, making the United States one of the most af- fluent and strongest powers on earth. But it may also very well have made our country more sensitive to and ready for rebellion.

It must be kept in mind that rebellion is not always or necessarily undesirable. The Establishment and its institutions are slow to change, and often it appears that desperately needed change is precipitated only by the advent of overwhelming crises such as war or severe depression. Those who represent and support the status quo are al- most inevitably against any kind of *rapid* change in our culture. Nevertheless, the culture does establish barriers and when these bar- riers, which we suppose to be appropriate, conflict with human needs and desires, then some kind of reaction must occur. If this conflict results in a change for the better of the status quo, so be it. On the other hand, if those forces which stimulate rebellion against the Es- tablishment are primarily concerned with destruction of the status quo without a pattern for improvement, then only chaos can result. This should be avoided and halted, if necessary, by disciplinary means. Since it is difficult to keep our emotional biases from blurring our vision, we may not be able to see clearly a significant aspect of the problem—whether or not the change would lead to improvement. Is it possible to create a social system and educational institutions that have a built-in mechanism for change, so that these institutions never become outdated nor permit the devastating crises we are expe- riencing today?

We are now confronted with a rebellion from a number of minority groups; perhaps one of the greatest, if not *the* greatest, threat is that of racism—not only the traditional racism of white against black, but also the new militant racism of black against white. In the last year or so, we have seen evidence of increased racism by blacks against whites. I would define racism as a belief that one's own race is su- perior to another and in the use of a policy of enforcing that belief. But there are other minority groups (such as Mexican Americans, Puerto Ricans, and—of particular concern because they are less vocal —American Indians) representing grossly disenchanted groups whose problems must be dealt with.

In many respects the rebellion of a minority group may represent a maturational process. At first, for example, the demand of the blacks was for the right to privileges which whites had reserved for themselves. This has now, it seems, resolved itself into an ethnic identity crisis, as evidenced by the slogan, "Black is beautiful." It would seem wise to maintain a multiracial society with the true identity of each group preserved, but with cooperative and interactive functions. I feel that no rational person would deny that not only have many tragic attitudes and actions toward the blacks occurred in the past, but that they still persist. On every important campus in the country there are groups—some large, some small, some black, some white—rebelling against the educational status quo. And in many instances such action is appropriate.

Perhaps the most serious immediate need is to understand the problems which have been created for the black and other minority groups. It is necessary for those in control to cooperate in working out the best possible solution. In this connection I would like to quote recommendations of Michael Beaubrun (3) of Jamaica, who states that ". . . a program aimed at alleviating tensions between groups in conflict should have both short- and long-range goals." He describes the short-term goals as a kind of "brush fire" operation, and states that long-range goals should include such factors as:

(1) Adjusting gross economic injustices and providing freedom from economic anxiety. (2) Reducing the overall level of anxiety for the community as a whole. (3) Uniting the community in a common cause, e.g., substituting national goals for those of race or class. (4) Building the self-image of subordinate minorities by incorporating teaching about their cultural roots and history and their importance in the history books in schools. (5) A key factor is the importance of not allowing segregated schools to develop. Denominational schools all too frequently separate communities by separating children in their crucial developing years. (6) The use of unifying symbols, to enhance awareness of the community or nation as a group. (7) The use of legislative and political power to ensure that people "behave" in the desired ways.

Dialogue has been described as the gut-level exchange between adversaries speaking specifically for themselves to each other, a kind of confrontation which presumably will aid in communication between those holding different views, for example, between minority or ethnic groups and the Establishment; and violence has been described as a mode of communication which gets the message across more quickly and makes the point more emphatically. If this is a correct interpretation, we must strive to keep dialogue going and avoid the kind of communication which occurs from and through violence. On the other hand, dialogue will not succeed if the adversaries make impossible demands and will not accept any kind of compromise. In fact, compromise has become a dirty word in some groups.

The Black Caucus which met at the 1969 Annual Meeting of the American Psychiatric Association presented a list of demands, some of which were quite obviously impossible to fulfill in accordance with the Constitution of the Association. Fortunately, however, the leaders of the Black Caucus were cognizant of the difficulties and agreed to suggestions that were mutually acceptable, a healthy group interaction resulting in valuable developments. Unless confrontation leading to adequate dialogue and a significant improvement in the lives of minority groups—and a better understanding of their plight by the majority—can be achieved, the future looks very dismal indeed.

Group and mob philosophy being what it is, it is not difficult to understand how an attempt to improve a situation may often result in behavior getting out of hand and a completely irrational type of acitivity developing. One has only to remember what occurred at Columbia, Berkeley, other compuses, and Chicago to realize that constructive agitation for genuinely needed changes can be neutralized and negated by the overreaction of those who feel that the powers that be lack understanding of their needs.

Given the demand for technologic sophistication, it is easy to understand why technology has so far outdistanced sophistication in social action. In fact, I think we can all agree that sociologic developments involving interrelationships between individuals, communities, or nations are still in a relatively primitive and unsophisticated stage. Such sociologic development could be considered not only primitive but quite naïve in our present culture, and yet interrelationships, both individual and national, are based on the cultural patterns in which we live. Often technologic accomplishment seems to derive a good share of its motivation from fear; on this basis it would appear that the national economy in some respects also relies on fear for support.

This includes many factors—such as those involved in competition, in failure, and in what Henry (4), in his book, *Culture Against Man*, called "the great External Fear, the fear of the Soviet Union," and, I might add, of Red China. This he considers to be particularly significant in the stimulus for progress in various industries, such as automobile and aircraft. He states:

> In this, he [the self-employed] is little different from the worker because the protection the worker wants from his union is not only against low pay, insecurity and poor working conditions: what he also wants is a safe-guard against *humiliation* for that is spiritual murder. . . . All languages are deductive systems with a vast, truth-telling potential, imbedded in vocabulary syntax and morphology. Yet no language is so perfect that men may not use it for the opposite purpose. One of the discoveries of the 20th Century is *the enormous variety of ways of compelling the language to lie.*

I couldn't agree more. It is clear that many of the present-day television portrayals, as well as certain books and advertisements, are clear-cut manifestations of "the enormous variety of ways of compelling the language to lie." These distortions are not likely to be the major causative factor in youth unrest and militant dissent; yet, inevitably, they can serve as a determining factor and may, in certain instances, actually serve as a precipitating factor.

Regarding the rebellion of students, alienation is best described as a sense of detachment from the values regulated by society which, in turn, leads to nonconformist behavior. The dimensions of alienation have been described as powerlessness, meaninglessness, normlessness, and social and self estrangement. There may be, in my judgment, a small group of individuals who are causing difficulty—acting out their instinctual drives, as it were, in an immature fashion—simply for destructive purposes. It is difficult to correlate individual psychodynamic formulations with complex social phenomena. Therefore, it is not possible to vouch for the accuracy of a statement which has been made that some of the rebellion represents a kind of reliving of the oedipal situation, with the power structure symbolizing the father figure and the student trying to resolve his oedipal fantasies. On the surface, it is easy to rationalize the need for change, and I believe that there is little doubt that unconscious and irrational wishes which subsequently become rationalized under the guise of social idealism do exist in many individuals pressing for violent social change. It is necessary to realize that we cannot, in the final analysis, interpret with any degree of accuracy the behavior of a group in terms of individual dynamics, nor should we in turn use notions of individual psychopathology to argue away the need for change in many areas. More importantly, however, there is, I think, the much larger group of student rebels who philosophically are idealistic, and who feel a genuine need and a basic right to have some part in determining the purpose and content of their education and to overcome discriminatory practices encountered outside their idealistic group. Resulting behavior, of course, can easily get out of control, as it has.

In this connection it is interesting to consider the role of some of the faculty members who, in becoming too emotionally involved in such rebellions, stubbornly and strongly support the rebels whether the rebellions are rationally based or not. One is tempted to wonder about the maturational level of these faculty members. On the other hand, I would strongly support those who recognize the need for change, and who seriously attempt to understand this need and to help in controlling the changes, rather than trying to effect an impulsive and poorly thought-out action.

The other side of the coin is that, ruled as we are by our unconscious and often poorly controlled drives, it is easy for the Establishment to delude itself into feeling that it has been liberal when, in effect, all it is doing is repatterning its rigid, arrogant, and established self-perpetuating "territoriality." Such a reaction may, of course, create still more conflict. Although, according to Henry (4), culture appears to be based more on drives than on values, both are involved. There are many differences in our culture from the apparently simple culture of so-called primitive societies. If we analyze our culture, it is not difficult to assume that we are not far from our own primitive background.

Pinderhughes (5) is quoted as saying ". . . that a social order unresponsive to reason requires repeated crises for significant change." It is to be hoped that both the rebellious forces for change as well as the Establishment will direct some of their energies to self observation, which should diminish irrationally determined tendencies that turn dialogues into diatribes and lead to impulsive destructive behavior.

I can best conclude this discussion by referring to a statement of one of my friends who suggests that the "fight for freedom" is an unconscious quest for more discipline. As Hegel put it: "Freedom is the recognition of necessity." But freedom does not mean the opportunity for unlimited self or group indulgences without concern for the rights of others. It may be all to the good that the rebellious have idealistically resolved to fight against the corrupting influences of the power structure; but I submit that at the same time they should feel a deep moral obligation to do battle against contrasting tendencies within themselves. We need to check our own inner ambivalence and to guard against that which could be called mental contagion—the passive taking over of rebellion by inner compulsion and not by outer justification. Finally, let us guard against revolt against the laws of history, misunderstood tradition, and the genetic historical endowment which is a part of all of us. This would perhaps, in part, explain why freedom fighters try to destroy the very institutions on which they are dependent. Our institutions must recognize the errors which have been perpetrated and perpetuated. Sometimes this can be brought into general awareness only by a crisis. However, we do know that the most open and aggressive rebellion of an adolescent may be an unconscious demand for discipline; to be effective, such discipline must be appropriate and rationally determined. For centuries, in each generation there have been dire predictions made for the future. In each such situation the crisis has been resolved—sometimes well, sometimes poorly. Now, for the first time, the potential for mass destruction of the world as we know it exists. This may be the last opportunity appropriately to resolve present conflicts.

The young and militant of today are seeking more awareness, more opportunity to make their own decisions. Much of life experience is now cut and packaged like food at the supermarket. Nevertheless, most of us believe as I do, that there is still opportunity for creativity and accomplishment; but, unfortunately, it is not universally available. Thus, the so-called Establishment must speed up necessary changes so that there is, in truth and in fact, equal opportunity for all. This necessarily calls for reconsideration of our national values since values and value systems are the controlling factors in culture formation. We must understand our culture to understand why we as a nation believe as we do. We must as a nation—and quickly but not impulsively—be more concerned about societal factors than dollars, and invest more in the resolution of societal problems and less, if necessary, in technologic progress.

It behooves us all to hear the voices of dissent and to react to them appropriately—not in anger but in understanding and justice, with due respect for human rights and dignity. We inevitably seek answers but it would appear that an answer is not immediately available. Rather, institutions must be developed which will bring about the necessary changes through due but not slow process.

REFERENCES

1. INGLE, D. J., *Univ. of Chicago Mag.*, 41:28, May-June, 1970.
2. SPIEGEL, J. P., *Toward a Collective Theory of Violence,* unpublished address delivered before the APA Midwestern Divisional Meeting on Aggression and Violence, November, 1968.
3. BEAUBRUN, M. H., "Community Programmes for the Resolution of Group Tensions," p. 16, Paper read at the Seventh Caribbean Conference for Mental Health, Trinidad, July 27 to August 2, 1969.
4. HENRY, J., *Culture Against Man,* Random House, New York, 1965.
5. PINDERHUGHES, C. A., *Amer. J. Psychiat.*, 125:11, 1969.

12

Eschatology and the Ecological Ethic

EDWARD H. KNIGHT, M.D.

Clinical Professor of Psychiatry
Louisiana State University Medical School

In this brief rendition the proposition is offered, and examined, that survival of the human species as a human goal is not necessarily a sacrosanct guiding principle. More precisely, the automatic acceptance of such a principle or quasi-natural law as basic to all human thought and planning may in itself be detrimental and perhaps even a bit "crazy." The allusion to cultural insanity is not entirely facetious since the striving for species omnipotence has similarities to clinical paranoia. From this it would follow, clinically, that the human race may fare no better in its effort to replace God than did Freud's Schreber.

I always experience a certain naïve pique on hearing or reading, in the course of various scientific discussions, the resounding argument "clincher" that unless some one or other course of action is undertaken, the human race will not survive. Why should this, even if true, win arguments? Many scientific investigations seem to be directed more toward the discovery of new techniques for survival than toward pursuit of truth and understanding. What use, the advocates of applied science cry, is there for irrelevant information—sterile truths without useful application or adaptive advancement. (Knowledge for its own sake, that is, enjoyment, is passé.) This polemic has become even more forceful and urgent in the atomic age as scientists respond to the call for social responsibility. Ivory tower science is a dangerous luxury in a world threatened by self-destruction. The scientific community, it is said, must no longer remain aloof and should join the

87

mainstream of responsible political intelligentsia in steering our species toward eternal survival.

Man's awareness of his existence, while painful and a mysterious wonder, is not in itself sufficient explanation or justification for the notion that his species should or could survive indefinitely, or even that he must attempt this feat.

Regarding the need for relevance in science, social or otherwise, I would have no quarrel since this simply and correctly admonishes us that scientists should be educated persons and not merely technicians. However, the implicit assumption that educated scientists should have as their guiding light or *raison d'être et ouvrer* the battle cry, "homo sapiens in perpetuity," is definitely suspect.

It may well be that group or individual survival simply means avoidance of extinction. A better definition of survival might be the effort with each generation to redefine creative living. The guiding principle of avoiding death cannot be equated with learning how to live. In fact, overcommitment to the former may well lead to the loss of the latter. So great is man's fear of disappearance, annihilation, extinction, or death that he now regards all efforts to ward off the grim reaper—individually and collectively—as unassailably good, a strange paradox considering the performance of this murderous biped. Somewhere in this process the business of living has been lost amidst the struggle to avoid dying.

Otherwise enlightened scholars, usually professing a humanistic personal philosophy and no particularly recognizable religious bias, accept out-of-hand that the principle of perpetual species survival is not only biologically sound but philosophically beyond question. One cannot contest this or any other such declaration of faith, but one can certainly object to the inevitably accompanying "rider clause" which holds that the principle in question is logical and rational. The idea that homo sapiens ought to survive forever is as much a piece of unproven, "revealed" truth as is the story of Adam and Eve. No formal religion, save perhaps Thomism, would consider its acts of faith as objectively rational. The positivist may well, and as easily, demolish the humanistic assumptions of natural science as they have those of natural religion.

Perpetual species existence as an inviolable biologic tenet also seems open to question on biologic grounds. In fact, species change, disappearance, and flux seem more to reflect the course of evolution. Animals fulfill their functional destiny and survive if survival is their lot. Anthropomorphically speaking, they are more interested in their reflexes, territorial integrity, mating responses, and the fullest expression of their potentialities than in species perpetuation. Living out as fully as possible their constitutional imperatives, they defend, flee, and procreate, all with whatever passes for pleasure and satisfaction, hardly including the preservation of their own image ad infinitum. The whole matter of the tension between the individual animal's survival needs and his compulsive biologic mandate to reproduce is *not* understood! The so-called law of survival has never been demonstrated in the animal kingdom to have precedence over all other forms of creaturely activity, except perhaps in a most simplistic, individual manner.

To be the "chosen ones" either of God or biology is in effect starting off with a couple of paranoid strikes against us. The paranoid orientation may help for a time in the fight to survive, and does elicit a hostile confirmation of one's importance from a responsive environment. We (human beings) have set about to conquer (sic!) this hostile world of nature and are now seeing that the results of our divine conquests are consuming us. In turn, we vent our desperate exploitative rage on one another in typically paranoid fashion. Hopes for new worlds to conquer, that is, new paranoid targets in the celestial spheres, offer temporary relief from self-hatred and fear. Certainly, if we pollute the cosmos, we may also find enemies "out there" and happily continue our biologically paranoid battle for survival.

It is tempting to speculate on the sad consequences of misapplied Western monotheism. Judeo-Christian man has nurtured himself psychologically on the belief that his existence was made meaningful as an expression of a God who, in turn, had no significance other than that His children were the center of all His concern—a delusion permissible and even necessary for the infant vis-à-vis his parent— but fatal beyond the oedipal stage. This defining and explaining of all things, even first causes, in terms of oneself, is paranoid, and leads to a need to control last causes, that is, eschatology. Even the deity is defined, and certainly felt, as the God of man—not of existence. Man has not been able to tolerate the notion of a deity whose interest actually transcended man, a God of all being and existence. The hidden paranoid need to take over and assimilate the omnipotent

powers that both menace and endorse, persecute and love is clas-
sically paranoid, and all too reminiscent of Schreber who ended
dissolved in divine celestial intercourse. Society is not too far removed from this aspiration when it seeks to take over and control
the chromosomal mechanics of its own evolution. Here again, this
is not objectionable, but to do so blindly and solely to ward off
extinction and exalt a dubious self-image cries out for reconsideration.
Efforts to participate in the *creation of oneself* are suggestively symbolic of a massive oedipal effort not only to assume the father deity's
great power but to usurp his generative function in the primordial
bed of Mother Nature. Conservationists who protest the "rape of
nature" are suggestively symbolic here! The resemblance to paranoia
must be taken seriously.

Eschatology, we are told, deals with the dogma of final things,
the end of all, both man's experience and the unique happening called
man, and existence itself. Biologic and scientific philosophy claims no
interest or legitimate concern with eschatology—a disavowal which
cannot be accepted. Consciously or not, the philosophers of science,
being inescapably bound into the Western ethos, are the most bla-
tant and vigorous exponents of "man's survival above all." This has
been the wellspring of the scientific *Weltanschaung*. The ubiquitous
enmity of journeymen scientists toward philosophy may in part result from an unconscious wish to avoid exposure of their bandwagon
participation in the unedifying ethic of human survival at all costs.
Crudely put, the slogan "To Hell with nature and all else—man must
survive" is more crude, and even stupid. In mistaking the natural
impediments to the human "take-over" of the biologic world as enemies, the scientific community has partaken of Western man's paranoia. Scientific understanding has meant mastery—not blind mastery
for its own sake, which would have been better—but mastery in the
interest of vain, omnipotent, eternal survival.

Underlying this cultural motif is the desperate collective fear of
death and extinction of the self. We are as reluctant to face our
personal as we are our species demise, and fight the inevitability of
the former by striving to ward off the latter. To do this we must
assume the omnipotent powers of a deity whom we define as basically man-centered. Projecting his own fragile psychologic appara-
tus into this vain struggle, man changes his life mission from living
to avoidance of dying. All nature becomes his enemy as the quest is

vacuous. Every wave that rises to fall and every splattered roach reminds him of his finitude. Survival is his perversion, and his great talents for living are subverted into fouling his nest.

The conclusion is not that man cannot survive without tending his environment, but that he must shift from his narcissistic world view and values to an "ecological ethic." This implies that his values place him not as a splendid object in an inconsequential field, but as a piece of the whole, all of one cloth. He must somehow find a meaningful action-oriented stance toward "the fallen sparrow" somewhat more elevating than "I'm glad it wasn't me"; not as custodian or caretaker in the panorama of nature but as a fellow stockholder with more or less voting shares in comparison with other objects and aspects in the natural scene. It is not in directing a drama either toward or away from some desired or feared eschatological end, but in "getting it all together" with feeling and respect for all parts, that we dimly sense the ecological ethic. Perhaps the elusive orientation that I am suggesting may more closely resemble esthetic or artistic posture rather than religious or scientific. So be it; somehow it seems more comfortable and fitting to contemplate an existence of beauty and harmony than one that is holy or reasonable. This is the basis for an ecological value system.

According to an ancient Hebrew saying, God expressed the fervent wish that His people would attain grace (fulfillment) without Him; without Him as either protector or reward giver I would suppose, and even more important, without Him as an object of pathologic identification. Only by seeking to incorporate the omnipotent fantasies of God-like power over self, world, and existence could man have sickened into paranoia.

What way out? Assuming some plausibility for the argument that man has entered a cul-de-sac of fruitless paranoid seeking for a fantasied power that explains nothing and can only destroy himself, the way out can be only in making a fateful choice. He must choose either to cling regressively to the belief that he is the chosen object of his own perpetual worship in his own eternal world, or elect to accept his status as one of many valued objects of existence. What this calls for on the positive side is not known. Perhaps it may mean visiting the moon simply because it is there and we wish to study it, rather than getting there first with our missiles.

This may involve another of the famous humiliating dethronements in man's evolving concept of himself: from Copernicus to Darwin to Freud, and now the great denouement of the atomic age demonstrating the futile helplessness of man's efforts to control that which is uncontrollable, his final fate. He is not the premier Prince of Creation but only one of many creatures who may or may not survive. He must choose to live as fully, as richly, and as gracefully as befits the best equipped animal in the garden. If he wastes his energy in the blind pursuit of eternal omnipotence and survival, he will never live— even if he survives. If he bends his efforts toward humble harmony with the living biologic matrix, then he may or may not continue, but at least he will have lived well and not destroyed himself in vicious infantile rage.

13

Man and the Machine

ROBERT S. GARBER, M.D.
Medical Director, The Carrier Clinic

In an editorial on September 19, 1970, the *New York Times* commented with concern about the report that a Yale psychiatrist had implanted radio equipment in a chimpanzee's brain and had devised a technique permitting a computer to make specific changes in the animal's brain waves. While noting that the research is aimed at finding new techniques to help the mentally ill, the *Times* observed that it represents "at least a first step down the road toward the nightmare vision of a brain-controlled population." This editorial points up much that I, like many other psychiatrists and behavioral scientists, have been concerned with recently. The facts of the technological revolution are upon us. There is a vast potential for both good and evil in the new technological developments. As a psychiatrist I am particularly interested in how these developments affect people emotionally. I also feel strongly about the need for us to pause long enough to take a good hard look at where technology is leading us, for I fear that if we are not careful, we will have no alternative but to accept what the machinery gives us.

In this paper I will discuss some of the most significant recent technological developments, paying particular attention to their applications in psychiatry and other branches of medicine.

Ninety-five percent of all the scientists the world has ever known are alive and working today. The acceleration of their learning and the new knowledge they will gain and materials they will produce in

Delivered at the Arthur P. Noyes Memorial Conference, October 17, 1970, Philadelphia, Pa.

the next 50 years defy the imagination. In the United States we have developed a technological base so extensive and powerful that it has become a fundamental ingredient of our economic, social, and political decision making. It has brought us great capacity for industrial growth, employment, and national defense (1). It promises us a golden era of excursion into outer space and an efficient, high-energy civilization on earth where man can live with new economic security and with ample leisure time. Central to this technological giant, which some may call a monster, is the process of automation. Automation is taking over one area of human activity after another: war, industry, traffic, medicine, even politics; and the electronic computer is the ingredient basic to successful automation.

The scientific revolution has resulted in a number of assaults on man's egocentric conception of himself. Copernicus showed that our world is not the center of the universe, Darwin showed that man is part of the same evolutionary stream as animals, and Freud showed that man is not fully the master of his own mind. The emergence of the computer may well be another such challenge to man's self-concept (2).

THE QUESTIONNAIRE

But before getting into the subject of computers I would like to touch on one of the forerunners of computerized methods, the questionnaire. In view of the increasing demand for medical care it became necessary to conserve the time and work involved in collecting, organizing, recording, and retrieving the data required for both medical practice and research. Questionnaires have never been generally regarded as substitutes for the personal, doctor-patient, history taking interview, but they have been recognized as having certain advantages. They save professional time while allowing the patient sufficient time to reflect and to answer the questions at his own pace; they remind the patient of certain emotions, conflicts, or symptoms that he might otherwise repress or suppress during the interview; they can highlight certain areas that may be overlooked during the interview at a time when the patient may be presenting a host of symptoms and complaints; and finally they provide clues, or even a full agenda, for the direct interview.

There are, of course, disadvantages. The static format may interfere with spontaneous changes of orientation and focus that take place in the personal interview. Also, questionnaires are geared to the average examinee, leaving little leeway for patients who do not conform to this average. Furthermore, it is not possible to ensure that all questions are really understood and thus properly answered.

However, the main objection to questionnaires, and to computers, as aids in history taking and diagnosis is the possibility that they may interfere with the doctor-patient relationship—or, in psychiatry, with establishing a working rapport or transference relationship. Of course many factors, originating on both sides, affect the interactions between doctor and patient. They include the patient's social, cultural, and ethnic background and the nature of his illness, particularly his emotional condition, on the one side, and the physician's background, training, and specific orientation on the other. The wide variety of these factors accounts for the fact that no conclusive and encompassing concept for the doctor-patient relationship has been formulated. On balance, it may be assumed that the information obtained from questionnaires may be more valuable for diagnosis and preparing for future therapeutic action than the additional time that would otherwise be consumed in initial direct interviews. The questionnaire and its descendant, the electronic computer, are here to stay.

THE COMPUTER IN MEDICAL SCHOOLS AND HOSPITALS

Virtually every major medical school and hospital is either experimenting with the application of the computer to a medical or hospital problem area or is making plans to do so. Computer and medical equipment manufacturers are devising new hardware and hospital applications. In order to reduce costs and to step up the efficiency of internal fiscal management, hospitals, of necessity, are turning to the computer. Computerizing the accounting and billing is the first stage. The next step, in part dictated by the shortage of trained nurses, is to assist in patient management and monitoring. Assistance with patient history taking and printouts of patients' records and nurses' and doctors' notes have already been undertaken in some hospitals. This may be followed by limited assistance in diagnosis and treatment. As medical knowledge is reorganized and the mass of experimental data not previously fully available to all of the medical profession becomes computerized and easily and widely available, the impact of the computer will become increasingly formidable. In about five years progress should be so advanced that a substantial effect will be felt in office and hospital practice. In about 15 years this effect should be widespread and profound.

THE COMPUTER AND THE INDIVIDUAL PHYSICIAN

Because of the costs involved and the probable resistance of the individual practitioner to the computer, the early impact will probably be more upon hospital than upon office practice. With increasing sophistication of equipment and programming it is inevitable that the individual practitioner will be forced to rely to a greater extent than before on the hospital, its equipment, and its staff in assisting in diagnosis and treatment of his patients. Certainly the economics of automated testing equipment may make the hospital the preferred setting.

As soon as it has been clearly demonstrated that the computer can cut down error in diagnosis and treatment, it will tend to attract the conscientious practitioner. For the same reason, malpractice insurance carriers may also force the individual practitioner to cut down potential malpractice claims by requiring judicious use of the computer as a prerequisite to coverage, or they may establish higher rates for those who do not enlist the aid of the computer. Accordingly, I can foresee that 15 or 20 years from now the physician's office may be hooked up either to a hospital or a medical school computer center, or in or close to a hospital or other institution offering computerized services. Hospitals in small cities will be connected by telephone to computers at large hospitals or medical schools. It is only a question of time until the average medical practitioner will be relying upon computers in his daily practice of medicine.

LOSS OF PRIVACY

Where is this new technology leading us? Will man achieve the understanding and capability to identify its dangers and make it work for the betterment of our human environment? Or will he become subordinate to the machine and lose his capacity to control these changes? It is clear that the effects of technological change on the individual and his feelings are varied. For example, we are often told that today's individual is alienated by the vast proliferation of technical expertise and complex bureaucracies, by a feeling of impotence in the face of "the machine," and by a decline in personal privacy (3). It is probably true that the social pressures placed on individuals today are more complicated and demanding than they were in earlier times. Increased geographical and occupational mobility and the need to function in large organizations impose difficult demands on the individual to conform or "adjust." It is also evident that the privacy of many individuals is encroached upon by sophisticated eavesdropping and surveillance devices, by the accumulation of more and more information about individuals by governmental and private agencies, and by improvements in information handling technologies such as the proposed institution of centralized statistical data banks. There is little doubt that the power, authority, influence, and scope of government are greater today than at any time in the history of the United States. But, as Professor Edward Shils points out in his study on technology and the individual, there is another aspect that we need to consider. First, government seems to be more lacking in confidence today than ever before. Second, while privacy may be declining, it does tend to decline in a sense that most individuals are likely to approve. For example, the average man probably "enjoyed" much more privacy in Victorian times than he does today. No one cared very much about what happened to him: he was free to remain ignorant, starve, fall ill, and die in complete privacy. Compulsory universal education, social legislation, and public health measures—indeed, the very idea of a welfare state—are all antithetical to privacy in this sense, but it is the rare individual today who is loath to see that kind of privacy go.

It is not clear that technological and social complexity must inevitably lead to reducing the individual to a "mass" or "organization" man. Economic productivity and modern means of communication allow the individual to aspire to more than he ever could before. Better and more easily available education not only provides him with skills and the means by which his individual potential develops, but also improves his self-image and his sense of value as a human being. This is probably the first age in history in which such a high proportion of people have felt like individuals. For example, no eighteenth century English unskilled worker, so far as we know, had the sense of individual worth that underlies the demands on society of the average resident of the black ghetto today. The range of individual choice and action today, all the way from consumer behavior to political or religious allegiance, is greater than in previous times.

The use of electronic high-speed computers on a large scale in hospitals, industry, and elsewhere throughout the nation has raised a number of fears. Not the least of these is the nightmare spectre of Orwell's 1984 that lurks within a computerized, programmed, classification dominated, machine controlled world. Within the last five years a great deal of controversy has arisen over the invasion of privacy and the possibility that computer technology will create a 1984 Orwellian-style world. Fears have begun to develop that machines will take over and that individual privacy and freedom will decrease. These fears have been strongly expressed by many organizations and citizens, and especially by the younger generation.

Some of the fears are justified. For example, congressional committees have been concerned about the invasion of privacy that might occur or be made easier by the creation of national data centers covering all people. Congressman Gallagher of New Jersey, Senator Ed Long of Missouri, and Mr. Vance Packard in various publications have all expressed concern over the possibility that Orwell's 1984 is creeping up on the American public (4). Fears have been expressed that a national credit information utility, which began to take shape in 1966 and which eventually could lead to the checkless-cashless society, would invade the financial privacy of every citizen. In 1967 Senator Long's administrative practice and procedure subcommittee held a series of hearings on the subject of computer privacy, during which several prominent scientists testified. In June 1969, an article surveying the subject listed 69 articles and books on the invasion of privacy and computers. One of these articles recommended a computer Bill of Rights that would help to guarantee privacy in computer-based data files (5).

ADAPTING TO CHANGE

Although such hazards of a machine society are unquestionably new, it must not be assumed that man has not experienced such fears before. With varying degrees of explicitness many persons have sought, since the time of Marx at least, to call man's attention to the shift away from naturalistic values implicitly required by machine civilization. As man was released from nature's grasp by his power-multiplying and labor-extending artifacts, he came under a new yoke; the man/machine interface had its own set of action priorities and behavioral imperatives.

Effective interaction with machines necessitated shifts in attitudes and changes in values. Nowhere has this been more evident than in the workplace. The utilization of steam power, for example, clearly implied the clustering of workers about factories. The accompanying value shift requirements have been noted, for example, by Elton Mayo, in his contrast of the "established" and the "adaptive" society (6). Clearly, the attitudinal skill most valued by modern industrial society is adaptiveness. Where the only constant is change, ready accommodation to change is valued behavior. To keep one's emotional equilibrium is not easy among the shifting patterns in which most of us live. One way to maintain a semblance of equilibrium will be to meet invention with invention—to design new personal and social change regulators. Thus, we need neither blind acceptance nor blind resistance, but an array of creative strategies for selectively shaping, deflecting, accelerating, or decelerating change. The individual needs new principles for pacing and planning his life, along with a dramatically new kind of education. He may also need specific new technological aids to increase his adaptivity. Society, meanwhile, needs new institutions and organizational forms, new buffers and balance wheels.

More important, the rate of change has been so great, the pace is now so forced, that a historically unprecedented situation has been thrust upon us. We are not asked, as the primitive Manus were, to adapt to a stable and dominant new culture, but to a blinding succession of new temporary cultures. This is why we may be approaching the upper limits of the adaptive range. No previous generation has ever had to face this test. Yet despair is not merely a refuge for irresponsibility. It is unjustified. Most of the problems besieging us stem not from implacable natural forces but from man-made processes that are, at least potentially, subject to our control. As every first-year student of anthropology knows, thanks to Margaret Mead, the Manus of the South Pacific emerged unscathed from the Stone Age into the twentieth century within a single generation—a seeming miracle of cultural adaptation. This success story of the Manus is often cited as evidence that we in the high technology countries will also be able to leap to a new stage of development without the undue hardship of culture shock.

We must recognize, however, that our situation, as we speed into the superindustrial era, is radically different from that of the Islanders. During the next 30 or 40 years we must anticipate not a single wave of change but a series of terrible heaves and shudders. I am speaking in a metaphorical sense but I fear that these disruptions may also occur in the literal sense if the violence of our times is any forerunner of things to come.

"FUTURE SHOCK"

And yet culture shock is comparatively mild in comparison with what Toffler (7) calls "future shock," a term coined to describe the shattering stress and disorientation induced in individuals subjected to too much change in too short a time. Fascinated by this concept, Toffler spent five years visiting scores of universities, research centers, laboratories, and government agencies, reading countless articles and scientific papers, and interviewing literally hundreds of experts on different aspects of change, coping behavior, and the future. Nobel prizewinners, hippies, psychiatrists, physicians, businessmen, professional "futurists," philosophers, and educators alike gave voice to their concern over change, their anxieties about adaptation, and their fears about the future. Toffler reports that he came away from this experience with two disturbing convictions: First, it became increasingly clear that future shock is no longer a distantly potential danger, but a real sickness which increasingly large numbers already have. This psychobiologic condition can be described in medical and psychiatric terms. It is the disease of change. Second, he gradually came to be appalled by how little is actually known about adaptivity, either by those who call for and create vast changes in our society or by those who supposedly prepare us to cope with them. In the most rapidly changing environment to which man has ever been exposed we remain pitifully ignorant of how the human animal copes (7).

Almost invariably, research into the effects of change focuses on the destinations toward which change carries us, rather than on the speed of the journey. The rate of change has implications quite apart from, and sometimes more important than, the directions of change. Any attempt to define the content of change must include the consequences of pace itself as part of that content. Future shock, then, is the dizzying disorientation brought on by the premature arrival of the future, and may well be the most important disease of tomorrow. It will not be found in a medical dictionary or in any listing of psychologic abnormalities. Yet, unless intelligent steps are taken to combat it, millions of human beings will find themselves increasingly disoriented and progressively incompetent to deal rationally with their environments. The malaise, mass neurosis, irrationality, and free-floating violence, already apparent in contemporary life, are merely a foretaste of what may lie ahead unless we come to understand and treat this disease (7).

On the one hand, the vast majority of our population, including educated and otherwise sophisticated people, find the idea of change so threatening that they attempt to deny its existence. On the other hand, there is the danger that those who treasure the status quo may seize upon the concept of future shock as an excuse to argue for a moratorium on change. Not only would any such attempt fail, triggering even bigger, bloodier, and more unmanageable changes than any we have seen, but it would be moral lunacy as well. By any set of human standards, certain radical social changes are already desperately overdue.

It is sometimes said that one hazard of the future—with the drive toward mass production, mass media of communication, and mass entertainment—is the death of individuality. But I am more optimistic than some. We have been told so often that we are heading for faceless uniformity that I think we fail to appreciate the fantastic opportunities for individuality that the superindustrial revolution brings with it. The Cassandras who blindly hate technology and predict an antheap future are still responding in knee-jerk fashion to the conditions of industrialism. Yet this system is already being superseded (7). A new freedom may come, not in spite of the new technology, but very largely because of it. For if the early technology of industrialism required mindless, robot-like men to perform endlessly repetitive tasks, the technology of tomorrow will take over precisely these tasks, leaving for men mainly those functions that require judgment, interpersonal skills, and imagination. Super-industrialism requires, and I hope will create, not identical "mass men," but people richly different from one another—individuals, not robots (7).

THE POSSIBILITIES

The human race, far from being flattened into monotonous conformity, will become far more diverse socially than it ever was before. The new society, the super-industrial society now beginning to take form, will encourage a mosaic pattern of evanescent life styles.

In their fascinating book, *The Year 2000*, Kahn and Weiner list one hundred technical innovations they think are likely to be effected in the last third of the twentieth century. These range from multiple applications of the laser to new materials, new power sources, new airborne and submarine vehicles, three-dimensional photography, and "human hibernation" for medical purposes. Similar lists are to be found elsewhere as well. In transportation, in communications, in every conceivable field and some that are almost inconceivable, we face an inundation of innovation. In consequence the complexities of choice are staggering.

This is well illustrated by new inventions or discoveries that bear directly on the issue of man's adaptability. A case in point is the so-called "Oliver" (on-line interactive vicarious expediter and responder). This is being developed to help us deal with decision overload. In its simplest form Oliver would merely be a personal computer programmed to provide the individual with information and to make minor decisions for him. At this level it could store information about his friends' preferences for manhattans or martinis, data about traffic routes, the weather, stock prices, and the like. The device could be set to remind him of his wife's birthday and even to order flowers automatically. It could renew his magazine subscriptions, pay the rent on time, and order razor blades.

However, some computer scientists see much beyond this. It is theoretically possible to construct an Oliver that would analyze the content of its owner's words, scrutinize his choices, deduce his value system, update its own program to reflect changes in his values, and ultimately handle larger and larger decisions for him. Thus, Oliver would know how its owner would probably react to various suggestions made at a committee meeting. In fact, meetings could take place among groups of Olivers representing their respective owners without the owners themselves being present. Indeed, some "computer-mediated" conferences of this type have already been held by the experimenters. Oliver would know, for example, whether its owner would vote for candidate X, whether he would contribute to charity Y, whether he would accept a dinner invitation from Z. In the words of one Oliver enthusiast who is a computer-trained psychologist: "If you are an impolite boor, Oliver will know and act accordingly. If you are a marital cheater, Oliver will know and help. For Oliver will be nothing less than your mechanical alter ego." Pushed to the extremes of science fiction, one can even imagine pin-size Olivers implanted in baby brains and used to create living—not just mechanical—alter egos.

Another technological advance that could enlarge the adaptive range of the individual pertains to the human I.Q. and its artificial manipulation. Widely reported experiments in the United States, Sweden, and elsewhere strongly suggest that we may, within the foreseeable future, be able to augment man's intelligence and information handling abilities. Research in biochemistry and nutrition indicates that protein, RNA, and other manipulable properties are in some still obscure way correlated with memory and learning. A large-scale effort to crack the intelligence barrier could pay off in a fantastic improvement of man's adaptability (7).

MAN'S ALTERNATIVES

Before accepting these so-called advances, we need to stop and consider the consequences and alternatives. Do we want a world peopled with Olivers? When? Under what terms and conditions? Who should have access to them? Who should not? Should biochemical treatments be used to raise mentally defective persons to the level of normal persons? Should they be used to raise the average? Should we concentrate on trying to breed super-geniuses?

On the other hand, it is also necessary to ask ourselves whether we really would prefer to return to the traditional condition of man in which each individual presumably related to the whole personality of a few people rather than to the personality modules of many. Traditional man has been so sentimentalized, so cloyingly romanticized, that we frequently overlook the consequences of such a return. The same writers who lament fragmentation also demand freedom—yet overlook the "un-freedom" of people bound together in totalistic relationships.

Even babies become aware early of the temporary nature of human ties. The nanny of the past has given way to the baby-sitter service that sends out a different person each time. The same trend toward time-truncated relationships is reflected in the demise of the family doctor. He did not have the refined, narrow expertise of the specialist, but he did have the advantage of being able to observe the same patient almost from the cradle to the coffin. Today the patient doesn't stay put. Instead of enjoying a long-term relationship with a single physician, he flits back and forth among a variety of specialists, changing these relationships each time he relocates to a new community. Even within any single relationship the contact becomes shorter and shorter. In my opinion the impact that this fragmentation and contraction of patient-doctor relationships has on health care ought to be seriously explored.

Is there some way to explain the scene without recourse to the fading jargon of psychoanalysis or the vague and murky clichés of existentialism? A strange new society is apparently erupting in our midst. Is there a way to understand it, to shape its development? How can we come to terms with it? The solution or, better, solutions —for I am convinced that there is no one royal road to man's destiny—lie in the burgeoning wisdom that experience will teach us. I am convinced that we must know more about man before we can hope to extract the maximum benefit from the machines he has created. Neither God alone nor machines alone will give us the answers. In the words of Alexander Pope, "Know then thyself; presume not God to span; the proper study of mankind is man."

REFERENCES

1. MUSKIE, E. S., "The Challenge of the Technological Revolution," in *Impact of Science on Society*, Vol. 19, No. 4, 1969.
2. LEE, R. S., *Public Opin. Quart.*, Vol. 34, Spring, 1970.
3. MESTHENE, E. G., "Some General Implications of the Research of the Harvard University Program on Technology and Society," *Harvard University Program on Technology & Society*, Reprint No. 8, October, 1969.
4. SPRAGUE, R. E., *Computers and Automation*, Vol. 19, Jan., 1970.
5. HOFFMAN, L. G., *Computing Surveys*, Vol. 13, March, 1970.
6. ERICSON, R. F., *Acad. Management J.*, Vol. 13, March, 1970.
7. TOFFLER, A., *Future Shock*, Random House, New York, 1970.

14

How Private Is Privacy?

HERBERT C. MODLIN, M.D.

Director, Department of Preventive Psychiatry;
Director, Division of Community Psychiatry
The Menninger Clinic

In these times of swollen populations, of elbow-to-elbow and bumper-to-bumper living, privacy has become a precious essence. To ask, "Are we losing our privacy?" is naïve; more appropriately one might ask, "How much and how fast?" Technologic snooping (long-range camera, hidden microphone) and psychologic prying (polygraph, psychologic tests) are not the only accepted methods of inquiry by government agencies, industries, and individual citizens.

Several cities are experimenting with consolidated, computerized public records, including vital statistics from birth, marriage, divorce and death certificates, as well as information from the public school system, police department, public health office, draft board, tax department, newspaper vaults, court records, bank deposits, security investigations, church membership, automobile register, real estate files, and other sources. The touch of a button can produce for scrutiny this full array of data concerning any citizen—and without his knowledge or consent.

Within the context of an imminent goldfish-bowl society, medical beliefs and attitudes concerning privacy, confidentiality, and privileged communication invite thoughtful re-examination.

The principle of confidentiality in medicine is based on two assumptions: (1) The patient's unreserved candor is necessary to the physician's optimally serving his needs; withholding of information by the patient can lead to erroneous diagnosis and erroneous treatment.

(2) In an atmosphere of complete trust and guaranteed privacy, the patient will reveal all—for his own advantage.

The maintenance of confidentiality is a professional burden, a special ethical responsibility the average citizen is not expected to assume regarding his fellow man. The physician, himself in part an "average citizen," may need occasional support, frequent reminders, and even the threat of reprisal to help him safeguard the confidences entrusted to him. Learning to keep confidences is an important lesson the professional teacher imparts to pupils; it forms one of the subtle rituals of our guild.

We are aware that absolute confidentiality is seldom possible, and are familiar with many encroachments "in the public interest." We are required to report communicable diseases, particularly venereal diseases, which may set in motion a variety of investigations, not only of the patient but of his associates and intimates too. We are accustomed to requirements that we report medical disability related to possible criminal behavior; e.g., gunshot wounds, knife stabs, and possession of narcotics. In many states, we are now allowed, or even required, to report not just the facts but even our impressions when suspicious of the battered child syndrome. A 1967 Massachusetts law requires physicians to report all habitual drug users, not merely those using narcotics but any drug the taker has become dependent upon—even aspirin.

We increasingly participate in third party problems: the obligation to disclose diagnosis, treatment, prognosis, or nature of disability for insurance applications, Social Security, Medicare and Medicaid payments, and other documents protecting public interests. In my state, we must report names and diagnostic labels of all psychiatric patients admitted to both private and public hospitals. And the end is not in sight!

These successful inroads into strict confidentiality may cause us to feel somewhat beleaguered; and we may anticipate that the feeling will grow. We are under greater pressure to justify and confirm the confidentiality of the doctor-patient relationship; occasionally our patients exert this pressure. Some evidence suggests that the psychiatrist is more concerned with problems of privacy than his patient. Many people, our friends as well as our patients, chatter about their secrets with abandon. We have had long experience with patients who voice no objection to being interviewed in a case conference;

to having their psychotherapy sessions tape recorded; to participating in expressive, uncovering psychotherapy before closed circuit television, the video-tape camera, or the one-way vision mirror.

In a narrowly semantic sense, I submit that people generally are less uneasy about sharing secrets than about avoiding shame, censure, embarrassment, ridicule, and guilt. Their concern is that private information will be used to affect their marital, parental, economic, legal, or social interests adversely. It is not the invasion of absolute privacy which disturbs them—we all need confidants. It seems that potential misuse of private information to accomplish public discomfort or injury becomes the practical issue.

Another issue: We must consider that we work with a kind of patient who is different from those seen by Hippocrates or even those of our country-doctor grandfathers. Today's average patient is said to be relatively literate, sophisticated, informed, and possessed of a respectable layman's knowledge of modern medicine. Commonly, having no family physician, he selects his own specialist to consult after making his preliminary self-diagnosis. He compares the treatments he receives with those described in the lay literature or by his friends; and he complains, sometimes through a malpractice suit, if he is dissatisfied with doctors' efforts.

It has been suggested that this new breed of patients is competent to participate in certain medical decisions, to bear part of the responsibility for medical consequences. The recent "informed consent" judicial decisions indicate that the patient's sovereignty over his own body and his own life now has considerable legal sanction.

Thus, the maintenance of confidentiality falls largely to the physician, with some legal support; patients really seem somewhat indifferent. Our conviction of the medical importance of privacy is based upon historic tradition, long clinical experience, and accumulated data. We are the experts in this regard—experts on psychiatric treatment and on the professional climate necessary to the conduct of good treatment.

Yet our patients, with increasing frequency, request relaxation of secrecy whenever they have other interests which will be served by disclosure. To what extent, then, should our judgment prevail in disregard of the patient's wishes? Here we risk the charge of professional arrogance—"The doctor knows best." Often he does, but does he always? How much should we honor the patient's privilege to exercise good or poor judgment in pursuit of his own autonomy, his personal freedom? A psychiatrist wrote recently, "The psychiatric tradition is that it is not necessary to follow a patient's wishes concerning divulgence of information regarding himself." This statement which most of us may approve most of the time is just the sort of pronouncement now recurrently being attacked. Can we vindicate it, not with aloof dignity, but with evidence which will persuade enlightened laymen?

In a recent newspaper article entitled, "To Hell With Medical Secrecy!" a science writer suggests that the previous traditional secrecy may be outmoded in our society. He says, "I am not, of course, advocating that doctors should be free to indulge in malicious or frivolous gossip about their patients and, in any case, the law provides a remedy for anybody who may find himself injured in such fashion. I am suggesting that the public should accept the idea that free and responsible use should be made of the immensely valuable information that every practicing doctor accumulates during every working day.

"Proper records analyzed by computer could well reveal the cause of coronary thrombosis and many other serious afflictions, and so point the way to their prevention. It could even reveal the people who ought not to be allowed to drive a motor car or have a seat in the Cabinet. Ah! But what about the sacred freedom of the individual? Freedom, my foot. We survive as a community or not at all; and doctors today are as much servants of the state as of their patients. Away with humbug and let us admit that all secrets are bad secrets. It is time we were shown for what we are."

In a similar vein both psychiatric and sociologic experts have decried the hypocritical and stultifying effects of traditional, unthinking insistence on privacy. The gist of their thesis is that privacy is a matter of guilt and shame. We feel we must keep covered such thoughts, feelings, and behavior as might be misconstrued or misused by others. In a "healthy" society, unburdened by a double standard (public stance versus private behavior), what do its healthy individual members need to conceal? With hypocrisy abolished, everyone's intentions manifest, is privacy a problem?

This argument can be but one side of the issue, but it is one side and cannot be casually shrugged off. Medicine can now less easily stand on its dignity, refuse to be questioned, and expect the time-honored "good old values" to carry the day. If we believe confidentiality essential to good medical practice, we must be articulate, prepared to defend our position rationally, ethically, convincingly.

We should differentiate the privacy of the patient and the privacy of the doctor. Occasionally it might be that our secrets—not the patients'—are threatened by exposure. The "informed consent" doctrine, for example, necessitates our revealing to the patient some of our thought patterns and manner of making prognostications; in short, our trade secrets. The physician may object primarily because he is uncertain that the patient's psychologic maturity and emotional stability are sufficient for his reaching medically sound conclusions; but the present legal tendency is to promote patients from the compliant, uninformed child level into the higher grade of participating adult. For better or for worse, part of the decision-making heretofore accepted as largely our professional responsibility is now being proposed as not exclusively medical at all.

Some of medicine's fierce defense of confidentiality may possibly be a hangover from a past reverence toward the mantle of the shaman, the anointed, the secret society, and the lodge brother aura. If it is, to any appreciable extent, this aspect of the "art and science" of medicine will be difficult to preserve.

I have presented a few issues concerning confidentiality and privacy from the viewpoint of the devil's advocate. If I were to extend this perspective into the mist beyond the horizon, I should suggest that as our creeping socialism accelerates to a gallop, as our population continues to explode, as urbanization becomes *the* way of life, as computers, records' systems, data banks, and multiple agency care increase, and as family functions give way more and more to community functions, confidentiality and privacy may become quaint words in an obsolete vocabulary.

15

Marijuana Problem

NORMAN Q. BRILL, M.D.

Professor of Psychiatry
Center for the Health Sciences, School of Medicine
University of California, Los Angeles

The marijuana problem is a multifaceted one with many unanswered questions. Is the use of marijuana dangerous and, if so, in what way? Who are the people who use it, and why and how do they get started? Are present laws regarding possession and use of marijuana necessary and helpful or unnecessary and harmful? Many contradictory statements published in recent years have created confusion.

It has been estimated by the Department of Health, Education, and Welfare that approximately 20 million Americans, or about one eighth of the nonchild population, have tried it at least once. Surveys of college campuses and more recently of high schools and elementary schools indicate widespread and perhaps increasing use of the drug by the young as well as the old, and by all socioeconomic and occupational groups. A survey at the California Institute of Technology showed that 20 percent of the student body had tried marijuana. A study by Imperi, et al. (1) at Yale and Wesleyan revealed that 18 to 20 percent of the students reported having used hallucinogenic drugs one or more times (about one fifth of these had tried it only once) and Pearlman (2) reported that the use of marijuana at Brooklyn College was not uncommon. In 1967 the UCLA student newspaper publication, *The Daily Bruin,* did a random sampling that showed that 25 percent of the students questioned had used marijuana at least once and, of that group, 20 percent had used it seven or more times. More recently, Fort (3) found that in one large urban

110

school district 18 percent of seventh-grade boys and 12 percent of the girls had used marijuana, while corresponding figures in the twelfth grade were 41 percent for boys and 43 percent for girls.

It is hazardous, if not impossible, to generalize about the characteristics of people who use marijuana. It is fairly well recognized now that all types of individuals use it and that the impression held some time ago that its use was predominantly by hippies has been shown to be incorrect. A fairly sizable group has been characterized as the experimenters or samplers, which includes those who have tried marijuana once or twice out of curiosity or as a result of urging of friends. They do not constitute any significant social or medical problem. There are chronic users who have been referred to as "potheads" (and more recently, "heads") who use marijuana primarily as an escape from reality or as a means of making life tolerable. These users are dependent on the drug and resemble chronic alcoholics but are often more disturbed. A good percentage have severe personality disorders; some individuals are borderline or overt schizophrenics, many of them eventually presenting in psychiatric hospitals and clinics.

The question invariably arises about the role that marijuana smoking played in the development of their disorders or breakdowns. Hekimian's and Gershon's study (4) at Bellevue Hospital showed that 50 percent of drug abusers who were admitted had been schizophrenic before taking drugs. Only a small fraction of the sample, however, were marijuana users. Many of this group give histories of having used LSD and other drugs, such as barbiturates and amphetamines, which complicates determination of the cause of their psychiatric difficulties. Some of the original hippies fell in this group and there seems to be little disagreement that the group clearly constitutes a medical and social problem.

Another type of individual who uses marijuana and is not usually seen in medical facilities has been raised in the ghetto where use of marijuana is often a cultural norm. This group appears to be primarily a social problem.

Most marijuana smokers fall within the group that uses it from less than once a month to every day, for relaxation, socializing, or getting intoxicated. It is this group that seems to cause the most concern and the least trouble. A large percentage of them are students. In many instances their parents are not aware of their use of marijuana and are shocked and frightened when they discover it. A varying but probably small percentage of the group mimic the hippie dress and behavior, or fall into the yippie group who are outspoken in their rejection of The Establishment. Most do not appear to be significantly disabled. They are functioning in school, work, or as parents. For the fairly regular user in this group there are various motivations. In some, especially the teenager, it is a way of rebelling against parents or The Establishment. Its illegality becomes a motivating force rather than a deterrent. For some it is an accompaniment of renunciation of the search for affluence and success. Some use it for temporary escape from reality, others seek mystical experiences or psychologic insights. Observation of the effects of marijuana suggests that it is often used to relieve underlying feelings of depression or anxiety.

While there is a seeking of increased awareness or sensual experience with music, colors, or beauty, the primary effects that are sought in the social users seem to be euphoria or feeling of well-being, relaxation, and a decrease in social anxiety. In a study reported by McGlothlin and West (5), in which the motivation for the use of marijuana was explored in 32 individuals who had used it 10 or more times, and in another study of a much larger sample by Keeler (6), euphoria and relief of tension were the most common effects reported. For those who are bored, it kills time. There has been a mistaken impression that marijuana is used extensively as an aphrodisiac, and that it intensifies sexual desire and pleasure. In some instances, when a couple anticipates a sexual orgy, they may use marijuana as others use alcohol to remove inhibitions.

An interesting effect of pot smoking is the sense of belonging developed by its users. They feel a kinship to one another that eases social intercourse even when not smoking. Pot smokers often maintain that it is more difficult to talk to someone who has not shared the experience and there is a good deal of recruitment. They can identify each other by manner of speech, much like two Americans in a foreign country who can spot each other and feel a great sense of kinship. There are undoubtedly many young people who start smoking pot in order to be one of the group.

A common response to question, "What does it do for you?" is "Try it." One girl said, "You can't describe the wonderful feeling to someone who hasn't had it any more than you can describe an orgasm to someone who hasn't experienced it."

Some pot smokers keep trying other drugs to see if they can improve on the experience or have a different experience, which is suggestive of experimentation in sex. One wonders if they are unable to feel real enjoyment or to find enough variety of enjoyable experiences. They appear to want relief from restraint and are impelled to do things that are forbidden or secret. Most students try marijuana from curiosity or social pressure, and many try drugs, including marijuana, for "kicks" or because it is the "thing to do." A common attitude is "why not try it?" The attitude is suggestive of "try anything," which can mean "let's not miss anything." In some it is an attempt to explore psychologic frontiers—to expand the mind—to get answers to life that religion used to satisfy. One opinion is that marijuana smoking is a manifestation of the new generation's exaggerated preoccupation with itself and its pleasures, that sexual experience is no longer the acme of sensual experience, and that it is searching for something even more satisfying beyond that. Different people react in different ways to the drug and there is great variation in amount and strength of marijuana.

Many aspects of the use of marijuana are not known: the extent to which users increase, decrease, or stop using the drug as time goes on; the extent to which protracted use produces dependence or passivity; and the exact nature of its physiologic effects. It is only in recent years that sophisticated studies have been undertaken. We do know that some individuals have adverse reactions and stop using it. One great unanswered question is whether those who manifest passivity use marijuana to achieve it or whether marijuana itself causes passivity. A related question concerns the dangers involved in its use. There was a time when anyone who used marijuana was believed to be well on his way to "going to the dogs." This obviously is not the case. However, if I had my choice—of someone I cared about using it or not—there is no question that I would prefer he did not. First, it is illegal; second, we do not know the effects of continued use; third, if used out of personal or psychologic need, rather than just experimentation, I would be concerned about the existence of the need as much as if the drug were alcohol or barbiturates; fourth, I have some concern about what else often goes along with use of pot, the renun-

ciation of worthwhile values and mores. This is admittedly a personal
bias.

For users who are functioning—as students, housewives, or in jobs—
there appear to be some characteristics, not always apparent, that
distinguish them to some extent from others. They are less likely
to have clear-cut life or occupational goals. They do not have the
same feeling about worthwhileness of life. They are more likely
to be against the war in Vietnam; intolerant of The Establishment
with its present moral and ethical standards; and less concerned with
religion; to be more pleasure-seeking, to look for new experiences, to
be more willing to take chances—including drug experimentation—
and less well adjusted.

Many have been concerned about use of marijuana leading to hard
drugs or narcotics. While some users have tried heroin, more have
tried LSD, amphetamines, barbiturates, and similar drugs. There is
insufficient evidence to substantiate the claim that marijuana is the
first step to drug addiction. It seems that many narcotic addicts start
with pot but very few pot smokers go on to narcotics (excluding the
very sick hippie group and the ghetto user). There is real concern,
however, that the professional basic suppliers of pot here and abroad
will mix heroin in with it, and that involuntary (and unknowing)
addiction might result.

WHETHER TO LEGALIZE

Fear has been expressed that legalizing marijuana would incur the
danger of more potent material being brought into the country. The
drug in use now (that is, grown in the United States and imported
from Mexico) is generally of low potency, certainly unlike the hashish
used in the Middle and Far East. There is great concern that if all
controls on marijuana were eliminated, potent preparations might
dominate the market.

The Committee on Problems of Drug Dependence (National Research Council) and the Committee on Alcoholism and Drug Dependence (AMA Council on Mental Health) took the position that abuse
of alcohol does not justify use of another drug, merely because it
does not cause cirrhosis of the liver or hangovers. It was pointed
out that comparisons between marijuana and alcohol are meaningless
unless dose and circumstances of use are considered. The amount

of marijuana most commonly used does not precipitate a hangover; but neither does the usual social use of alcohol. When advocates of the legalizing of marijuana claim that it is less harmful than alcohol, they are comparing the mild effects of marijuana at the lower end of the dose response curve with the effects of alcohol at the toxicity end of the curve, i.e., the "spree" use of marijuana versus acute or chronic alcohol poisoning. Alcohol is certainly a major problem; there is no point in having another drug replace or add to it. The AMA-NRC Committees maintain that if alcohol is bad for health, its use should be discouraged, rather than a substitute promoted, which, though not being narcotic, is habit-forming through producing a psychologic dependence. They have concluded that marijuana is a harmful drug, taking the position that although most Americans neither suffer lasting effects nor develop a strong dependence, there are nevertheless a significant number who do become chronic users with concomitant medical and personal problems.

While the percentage may be small, some young people who start using marijuana out of curiosity, thrill seeking, or the wish to be "in" with the group, proceed to experimental and spree-type abuse of other drugs, i.g., speed, STP, LSD, and the like. The relatively minor effects of weak marijuana preparations often give the false impression that any drug can be "handled" and a substantial number of young people are seen who are drug oriented, in addition to those who are strongly drug dependent, at the very time they are being called upon to make important career and other life-molding decisions.

Many users will deny that marijuana is habit-forming or that dependence develops, but the facts seem to be at variance with this. For some, the use of marijuana becomes a way of life that is not, and perhaps cannot be, easily given up; there are many instances where the use of pot has become an important way to maintain an escape from reality and in some, both LSD and pot are used. A great many disturbed adolescents are seen who have drug-taking in common, and one cannot help but feel that if they would or could stop taking drugs, they would benefit, and perhaps be able to solve their problems in more constructive ways.

An article in the May 17, 1967 issue of the UCLA *Daily Bruin* (7) reports that the bulk of the drug and marijuana traffic in this country (including the traffic on college campuses) is connected with organized crime. Only a small amount of marijuana is grown in flower pots. Even on the Pacific Coast most of the merchandise is supplied by the underworld rather than being smuggled across the Mexican border by independent agents. For example, one professional supplier on the UCLA campus is a clean-cut, middle-class student with law-abiding, upper middle-class parents; he has a B average. He deals mainly in marijuana, LSD, and methadrine; he can get "hard stuff" but doesn't want to. He purchases a kilo of marijuana for $40.00 (a little over $1.00 per ounce), cuts it into lids (one ounce) which he retails at $8 to $11 each. He sells exclusively to students. He receives his supply from a person who is one step removed from the mainline of supply in the intricate communications network of the organized narcotics ring.

The police, who are well aware of the criminal underpinnings of the marijuana trade, claim they are just trying to enforce the law. One factor that tends to create the hard line of the police is the antisocial attitude that many pot users have and so freely express. A reporter stated:

> The legal battle over marijuana is just a small skirmish in the much larger war between the mainstream of American society and a disaffected minority, mainly under 30. Marijuana has become for some a symbol of discontent with basic American values and with the goals and life styles of the older generation. Pot is their thing—as alcohol is for The Establishment. In some ways it seems to be a reflection of the impulse to test and sample all new and forbidden experiences. There is an increasing insistence on the part of the younger people that what they do—whether it be pot, sex, dress, et cetera—should be a matter of individual choice and personal normality as long as they don't harm anyone else. There are some who will insist the government has no more right to tell them what drugs they can or cannot take than it does to tell them what or how much food they can or cannot eat.

Most commonly, university administrators are not interested in prosecuting students who possess or smoke pot as long as they are not selling it. In one university, if a dormitory adviser reports marijuana in a student's room and the student admits it, no action is taken except to expel him from the dormitory, but not from the university. Administrations turn the other way; they are aware of prevalent use, but ignore it unless the use is forced on them.

The extent to which the use of marijuana in itself is causing problems for individuals and society is not known. It has been said that soldiers in Vietnam who smoke pot are more effective as a result and can tolerate their situation more easily. Certainly there are many misconceptions about its effect: it predisposes to crime, leads to taking hard narcotics, results in brain damage, and is like LSD. There is some suggestion that continued use of marijuana in large amounts leads to apathy and psychologic immobilization. Decrease in aggressiveness, competitiveness, and striving for usual goals are qualities that are sought after by some users rather than considered abnormal by them. If this is so, should society allow an individual to deactivate himself with drugs until he feels comfortable? What will the eventual outcome be? Will society have to take care of users? Already, many of the dropouts have applied for relief or unemployment insurance; some end up in jail, some have children who become wards of the State. In Keeler's study (6) there was an interrelation of high dosage, manifest schizophrenia, dropping out of school, and desire for psychotomimetic experience.

It seems likely that as long as we regard social maladjustment as illness, and consider the need for providing treatment in the same way that we do for a broken leg or pneumonia—that is, doing something to or for the sufferer—we shall have great difficulties, because sympathy toward the socially maladjusted is often mixed with disapproval and condemnation. The socially maladjusted person often insists he does not want treatment or sympathy. He has sought his pleasure by renouncing the usual cultural goals and often regards those who offer him help, like the psychiatrist, as being in need of help themselves. The dropout may regard himself as like the early Christians—like Christ himself—as the bearer of the true word that will save the world from self-destruction. Social illness or maladjustment needs a different kind of approach, one that regards an individual's fulfilling his responsibility to society, rather than the individual's immediate sense of comfort, as the minimal goal of treatment. Society will resent a person who, as a result of behavior that is known to be chronically self-destructive, does not support himself and becomes a burden on society.

How much of the concern about the use of marijuana stems from our general wariness about escape mechanisms, excessive dependence, and abandonment of self-control—behavior that creates problems not just for the individual but for those around him? Somehow there is concern that permitting each person to do what he wants—whether it be drinking alcohol, using pot, pursuing pleasure without restraint—is a regressive phenomenon that will shake the roots of our social structure. The anxiety created in society by those who insist upon "doing their thing" or "tuning out" is not totally out of concern for these persons. In part, it stems from unconscious envy and the attitude: "I do what is expected of me—why don't you do what is expected of you?" There is in everyone a latent intolerance of the restrictions and demands of society, and residuals of the wish to be taken care of, that appear to play a role. The Christian Ethic—love of one's fellow man, sympathy for the weak, and being one's brother's keeper —are goals that many strive for; but because people are human, they resent aggression whether it be active or passive. Love of one's fellow man is less possible when the burdens are felt to be excessive. Parents, at times, give up with regard to children who are beyond helping; wives with alcoholic husbands; husbands with chronically neurotic wives; and doctors with patients who can't be helped. Society rebels against people who can work but don't.

Lest we think the present state of affairs is unique in the history of man, Dr. Sidney Cohen (8) reminds us that there was an age of anxiety in nineteenth century England, when there was a great searching for a utopia or tranquility. It gave rise to a turning to opium, as exemplified by Coleridge, De Quincey, Poe, and others who sang its praises. The creativity of these men was not connected with the use of opium—it preceded it—and each one later turned against the drug. Coleridge called it "an accursed habit, a wretched vice, a species of madness" and attributed his neglect of his family and his deterioration to its use.

I do not suggest that marijuana is addicting, as opium is, but echo Cohen's reminder that new psychochemicals or drugs are likely to be overvalued and misused, especially during periods of heightened stress and frustration. How to enjoy life without euphoriants, tranquilizers, stimulants, and escapants is the question.

The laws prohibiting marijuana, like those against alcohol in the 1920s, have not significantly diminished its use. Under federal law, sale or importation incurs a minimum sentence of five years for a first offense, while first-offense possession brings a two-year sentence. This seems to be extremely severe for those who participate in occasional pot parties that are usually quiet, small gatherings of friends.

One individual arguing for legalization says, "It's more entertaining, cheaper, and cleaner than the movies, less degrading than alcohol, less dangerous than tobacco, and much more enlightening than television."

So the conflict and the arguments continue. I do not pretend to know the answers. There is much we need to learn—from research and from experience. It is clear that we need to distinguish between the effects of pot on personality, and the personality factors that preexist and are intimately related to the drug-taking. It is possible and even likely that the preexistent characteristics may become more pronounced with continued use of marijuana, but this, too, needs to be shown. For the time being, it is important to keep an open mind, a wait-and-see attitude, with the hope that research that is being pursued will provide answers that will permit a sensible, objective, constructive approach to the problem.

REFERENCES

1. IMPERI, L. L., et al., *J.A.M.A.*, 204:1021-1024, 1968.
2. PEARLMAN, S., *Drug Use and Experience in an Urban College Population*, presented to the 44th Annual Meeting of the American Orthopsychiatry Association, Washington, D.C., March 23, 1967.
3. FORT, J., *Psychiat. Opinion*, 5:9-15, 1968.
4. HEKIMIAN, L. J., & GERSHON, S., *J.A.M.A.*, 205:125-130, 1968.
5. McGLOTHLIN, W. H., & WEST, L. J., *Amer. J. Psychiat.*, 125:370-378, 1968.
6. KEELER, M. H., *Amer. J. Psychiat.*, 125:386-390, 1968.
7. J. T. P., *UCLA Daily Bruin*, 71:3, May 17, 1967.
8. COHEN, S., *Amer. J. Psychiat.*, 125:393, 1968.

16

Indochina: An Ethical and Professional Concern for American Psychiatry?

EUGENE B. BRODY, M.D.

Chairman, Department of Psychiatry
University of Maryland School of Medicine

Should a professional organization express a position on national policy when this policy concerns its area of special expertise? Is it the ethical responsibility of an organization of economists or sociologists or psychiatrists, for example, to speak out when the nation as a whole is affected? Is this not, in fact, the legitimate obligation of a profession? Where are the limits of such expertise when public policy issues are concerned?

The answers to these questions might be less difficult if the individuals making up such organizations could arrive at a consensus. Failure of consensus in a presumably scientific organization reflects both the limits of technical competence and the often unidentified factors which determine professional decisions. The professional acts of psychiatrists, while informed by science, are additionally determined by art, judgment, compassion, economics, feelings, and prejudice. Even the familiar acts of making a diagnosis or prescribing treatment are to some degree determined by hidden bias associated with social class. An opinion in court may be less a faithful reflection of science than of whether the doctor is employed by the defendant or the prosecutor.

Consensus is difficult enough in areas which have been traditionally regarded as the domain of medicine. Prevailing professional and public views of what is medically or morally permissible have undergone marked changes in accord with the evolving status of society and the role of the physician. In recent years industrialized Western nations have seen rapid modifications in attitudes toward drug usage, sexual behavior, the definitions and limits of pornography, sex reassignment surgery, abortion, contraception, and sterilization. Issues formerly regarded as the sole concern of public policy makers have become the explicit concern of psychiatry and medicine (as they once were in preindustrial eras when medicine men were acute social as well as individual diagnosticians). A stand on gun control has already been debated at length within organized American psychiatry. Unanimity of opinion has not been achieved, but the now accepted concern with violence, and the presumed connection of gun control with murder control, suggest that such unanimity may be near. The American Psychiatric Association, with no outcry from its membership, has already presented an *amicus curiae* brief arguing against capital punishment in a case which appeared before the Supreme Court. These examples of actions taken by our professional association are not immediately, although they are ultimately, relevant to questions of behavior and hence mental health. Further, they conflict with politically significant traditional values, for example, freedom to bear arms for self-protection; and appropriate punishment as a deterrent to criminals and an affirmation of the strength of social institutions.

Conversely, matters once regarded as the sole concern of medicine have entered the domain of public policy. Thus, in the name of public health the freedom of tobacco advertisers has been curtailed by law. Since this step has been taken in the face of powerful business opposition, it becomes altogether possible that liquor advertising and its impact on health and behavior will be the next focus of attention. These steps are congruent with those being initiated to reduce air, water, and earth pollution, with their already demonstrated health-damaging potential. Moves of this type which conflict with traditional freedom of business enterprise and have significant political implications suggest a reorientation of our national attitude toward health. United States values regarding the importance of the individual have stimulated a progression from the view that medical care (and implicitly health) is an individual privilege to one which declares it to be an individual right. The other (and not incompatible) view, implicit in the Soviet medical care system, is that a healthy population is a primary national resource and that health is not an individual's right as much as it is his obligation to society, that is, what society can legitimately expect from him in order to maintain its corporate strength. As our country moves toward its own amalgam of these views, combining individual rights with national needs, it is inevitable that the definition of health-relevant social factors will be an ever-broadening one. This projection of our social evolution evokes both hope and apprehension. Hope is for the development of adequate preventive measures which must include means for dealing with poverty, racial discrimination, exposure to occupational hazards, and other mediators of personal inadequacy, retardation, and ill health. Apprehension is for the loss of individual privacy and the gradual erosion of those privileges of self-determination and personal autonomy which we take for granted as part of being human. Both hoped for and feared eventualities involve ever closer relationships between clinical and public policy decisions.

When it comes to matters of international policy, especially those involving warlike confrontations with other countries, the diversity of opinions is even more marked. Some contributors to this diversity are territorial and deeply ingrained; they include fear of and fantasies about the unknown, retaliatory impulses in the face of threat, and the need to protect one's own home and family. Anxiety and anger are well-known disrupters of cognitive processes; they make long-term rational decisions extraordinarily difficult to achieve. Other factors contributing to conflicting opinions about government policy have components which are less obviously but, nonetheless, emotional. Many of these revolve around the question of information as it relates to the international posture of the United States. It is argued that overriding issues about which we know nothing determine our national policy. Some of these relate to developing military technologies. Others concern the alleged expansionist plans of other major countries. In the absence of crucial knowledge, which probably cannot be divulged for national security reasons, how can a professional association or its members take a foreign policy position based solely on health or ethical considerations? Our mental (or moral or economic or social) health, it is argued, cannot be the primary issue when our very survival as a nation vis-à-vis the threat of a foreign power may be at stake.

The nature and validity of presumed hidden information with such pervasive influence on national life, and of the decisions consequent to it, have recently met more extensive questioning inside and outside of government than ever before. Scientists and clinicians, more than ever before, are aware of the blurred borders between the provinces of technology and public policy. Medical organizations have not hesitated to take unequivocal positions of clear political significance when they sensed infringement on their rights, for example, to control the definition, use, and dissemination of "dangerous" drugs. They have even, as noted above, taken stands on politically significant issues not so clearly covered by their technical competence—stands which might be regarded as infringing on the rights of other organized groups. Yet they have devoted little explicit attention to understanding the historical shifts imposed by population growth, industrialization, and new technologies on the relations between professional-scientific and sociopolitical decision-making necessities and prerogatives.

Social change has especially blurred the boundaries between domestic and foreign policy decision-making. And nowhere are emotions more heated and opinions more divided than in the international relations and foreign policy area. This is why professional associations have not acted so vigorously on international matters with easily demonstrable effects on health and behavior as they have on domestic issues. They have simply not wished to fragment themselves over emotion-laden problems on the periphery of their ordinary concerns. On the other hand, none so far has tried to stop their members from expressing themselves as citizens with special expertise, that is, by identifying themselves as belonging to the organization. Thus, sociologists not wishing to divide their membership along lines of personal opinion did not deter their colleagues as individuals—identifying themselves as belonging to the American Sociological Association—from going on record in 1967 as opposing United States involvement in Vietnam. Within the American Psychiatric Association two extreme attitudes have been delineated. Some members wish a commitment to political action as such, utilizing the Association's status as a springboard, with no rationalization of the action in mental health or related terms. Others oppose not only action or organizational statements, but even the release of an opinion poll of the membership in reference to United States involvement in Vietnam. Their attitude is that such moves constitute political acts and a radical departure from the Association's professional and scientific aims. They are legitimately concerned with possible loss of the Association's tax-exempt status.

It seems likely that a significant number of psychiatrists stand somewhere between these two poles. They are not inclined to political action using the weight of the Association in the manner of any other pressure group. Nor are they inclined to prohibit the expression of opinion by colleagues identifying themselves as belonging to the Association and, therefore, as professionals in good standing. They are concerned, especially those working with youth, with the mental health impact of a war for which there is no broad popular support and which has so polarized the nation. They are impressed by the number of intelligent young people who see Vietnam as another reflection of parental failure and inconsistency and seem unable to find a middle ground, having as alternatives only violent protest on one hand or self-narcotization and retreat to a view that all is absurd on the other. They are impressed by the impact of the war on the poor and the black who are disproportionately employed in the fighting. They are sensitive to the degree to which even their conventional psychiatric decisions reflect changing social attitudes and personal bias and feelings. They are aware of the degree to which their own and other professional organizations have already taken politically significant stands on a variety of issues. They wonder if failure to recognize publicly the social-psychiatric impact of Vietnam will further alienate the present professional students who are future colleagues. Even those who insist that they prefer to work as private citizens for a cause they consider just find it difficult to disavow their status as professionals with special awareness of how changing social conditions influence the quality of American life and the mental health of its people.

These factors and many others make it difficult for psychiatrists to separate their attitudes toward domestic and international issues, and specifically Vietnam, from other social influences on family life and mental health. This is not to say that they attribute the current national malaise, many features of which have occurred at other times, solely to Vietnam. It is to say, however, that, surrounded by professional and social ambiguity and change, this middle group of psychiatrists is deeply troubled by the position in which it finds itself.

Too conservative to take action not explicitly informed by professional expertise or defined as part of their social role but unable to agree that as psychiatrists (though not as citizens) they should be muzzled regarding Vietnam, are they condemned to paralysis?

These psychiatrists may wonder if their Association would record itself as opposed to prejudice and poverty if called upon to do so. There is, fortunately, no need to make this pious affirmation since, Gunnar Myrdal's *American Dilemma* aside, it fits the national credo. Similarly, the Association appears ready to stand in official opposition to violence. But could it do so in respect to war? In the abstract this would undoubtedly be easier than to oppose a particular war, as many would-be conscientious objectors to Vietnam service have discovered. An organizational position on the particular, the concrete, or the temporal implies support or lack of support for elected policymakers and, hence, becomes political. Support for an ideal, however, transcends time and immediate circumstances and permits the organization and the politicians to join hands in public respect for the goal, safe in the tacit recognition that it cannot be achieved. Yet, as noted above, social fashions in morality and politics change rapidly, just as the brief history of modern psychiatry contains changing fashions in diagnosis and treatment. The general ideal of today presages the specific goals of tomorrow.

Scientists, in the wake of Hiroshima, have been struggling for a generation toward involvement in public policy decisions based on a conscious concern with the ethic of using the technologies which they have created. Many scientific leaders have come to feel it immoral and a retreat from their professional responsibilities to avoid ethical and policy positions. The positions, however, are based on systematic observations. They now refer to such specific social matters as the effect of U.S. involvement on South Vietnam's economy—or to specific biologic problems, such as the use of defoliants by the United States in Vietnam. Aside from the long-term ecologic impact of these latter, scientists question the ethics of procedures which, though laudably designed to save the lives of American troops, result in destruction of the food sources of deprived noncombatant populations.

Concern with rules of conduct and respect for life are embodied in the traditions of medicine. Yet practicing physicians have lagged behind scientists in their organized concern with the need to control the powerful consequences of technology for human ends. They have been even more cautious in their attitudes toward modifying the socioeconomic conditions behind so much ill health, although epidemiologic data would support them. Psychiatrists—physicians with special training in the sociopsychologic determinants of behavior and bodily function—would seem to have special responsibilities in this area where medicine, behavioral science, public policy, and ethics come together. As individuals they can no more escape recognition of the impact of the Vietnam war than of any other social condition upon the health and behavior of their communities and their patients. If as individuals, or banding together as American Psychiatric Association members, they wish to express opinions about or try to influence any aspect of public policy, including the Vietnam war, that should, in a democratic society, be their privilege, perhaps their obligation.

For the Association itself, as a supraindividual entity, is there also an obligation? This question is partly answered by what has already been written. First, the formation of national policy, even at the domestic level and in regard to clearly health-related matters, is uncertain, conflictful, and feeling-laden; at the international level it involves strong emotions which make dispassionate discussion extremely difficult. Second, rational programs aimed at ensuring individual and public health require attention to a broad range of policy questions, often far removed from the traditional concerns of physicians and psychiatrists. Third, the presumed scientific and objective decisions of psychiatrists are regularly influenced by unidentified emotional, cultural, and economic considerations. Fourth, scientists and professionals can no longer afford to ignore the ethical as well as the social consequences of their professional acts. Fifth, the boundary between professional versus political acts is no longer clear; reexamination of the criteria for tax exemption is both essential and probable. The Association, then, does have an obligation to facilitate and understand the process of decision-making about all issues bearing on health and human behavior. Facilitation and understanding require the freest expression of informed opinion from a variety of professionals and executives, the creation of new opportunities for data gathering and information exchange, and the highest degree of tolerance in all quarters, including government, for attacks on their emotionally important attitudes.

This essay is not a call for the Association to adopt a unitary position for or against the Vietnam war. It is, rather, a plea against ignoring issues by retreating into a self-deceptive attitude of scientific neutrality. As Boulding (1) has pointed out, in "the subculture of science . . . veracity is the highest virtue." If veracity, not neutrality, is the goal, the American Psychiatric Association's obligation is clear. It should encourage, through its committee and task force structure, an explicit examination of the ethical aspects and mental health consequences of pertinent governmental policy positions. If these consequences suggest support or disagreement with the policies in question, such conclusions should be published along with the data upon which they are based. In this way the American Psychiatric Association can retain its claim to being a scientific organization attempting to meet its ethical as well as its professional obligations.

REFERENCE

1. BOULDING, K. E., *J. International Affairs*, 21:1-15, 1967.

17

Mission to Russia

HAROLD M. VISOTSKY, M.D.

Professor and Chairman, Department of Psychiatry
Northwestern University

As the Soviet Plan is defined by the Ministry of Health, the principal goal is to improve and expand prevention programs. Although the level of understanding of psychiatric illness in the USSR is comparable to knowledge throughout the world, Soviet mental health programs emphasize a prevention approach.

The Ministry of Health places a high priority on properly located polyclinics, which are general medical clinics dealing primarily with early intervention and preventative programs, and these provide a wide variety of special resources in general medicine and psychiatry. The Russians take proper pride in the unique USSR system of neuropsychiatric dispensaries, their obstetric, pediatric, cancer and tuberculosis programs, and in the fact that their mortality rate is lower than in many other countries of the world.

There are nearly 600,000 physicians in the USSR, 75,000 of whom are oral surgeons and stomatologists, comparable to our dentists; this totals more than twice the number of doctors now practicing in the United States, and with 35,000 physicians graduating each year from the 82 Soviet medical schools, there are four times the number now graduating annually from American medical schools.

Medical school graduates in Russia are encouraged to spend at least three years in general practice before specialization. Postgraduate training is available in 13 new institutes with five postgraduate facilities. While the training courses offered in continuing education are brief—only three to five months—this program is successfully supplying current medical information to a great many physicians.

These postgraduate courses are stipend courses; the physician is on salary during his period of postgraduate education.

The Russian officials stated that when the number of physicians had reached a total considered optimal for the population, many of the present medical schools would be converted into postgraduate training centers with postgraduate training then becoming mandatory. In effect, they would continue to turn out the number of physicians necessary to replace those who retired or died, plus enough more to meet the needs of population increases; but beyond this goal, the primary mission of the medical schools would be to serve as postgraduate training centers.

This program also applies to the staffing of research institutes outside of medical schools, and these additional institutions presently number 300, but the Ministry plans still more such institutes for general intestinal, pulmonary, cancer and neuropsychiatric research.

On the fiftieth anniversary of the Russian revolution, the Soviets looked ahead to achieving a goal of a full range of medical services available to all citizens, and to the economic growth considered necessary to the fulfillment of this goal. Their goal is 700,000 physicians, or a ratio of one physician for each 400 citizens. The Minister of Health said the Russian people know their country places the highest priority on medical care and they encourage their sons and daughters to enter medicine. He envisions no problems in recruiting the additional students necessary to their plan; in fact, at the present time, medical schools are rejecting from four to 10 applications for admission for every acceptance.

Special recruitment advantages are offered within the field of neuropsychiatry. For example, although all medical personnel are given a one-month annual vacation, those serving in the mental health field are given two months of paid vacation each year. Women physicians, comprising 70 percent of the total, may retire at the age of 50 on full pension, and this pension is increased by 10 percent for those whose work was in the mental health field. Also, physicians working in this field receive some priority in the matter of housing.

A variety of medical specialties is desired and enlarged medical institutions with more multidisciplinary hospitals are envisioned. In cities, 1000- to 2000-bed hospitals are thought best for providing the variety of medical specialty services needed. In rural areas, regional hospitals of 400 to 500 beds are considered preferable for the same reason—these larger hospitals can best support the broadest profile of medical specialists and special services. Polyclinics in each area are planned in accordance with local or regional needs, but these plans are flexible, since the national government will match, but does not provide all of the necessary capital for such plans, once approved, and each area is expected to bear its share of the services it proposes to make available in the locality. The Soviets say they are able and willing to make medical resources equally available to rural and urban populations. Support of financial requests is based on service objectives, but it would be incorrect to believe autonomy exists; although the local government must show its willingness to support its share of the expense in providing the area with suitable services, the central government does the planning.

Proposals submitted are considered by the Ministry of Health, corrected and returned to the local republic for funding and implementation. However, the form of delivery of service does vary and some autonomy is allowed in meeting local needs. Russians emphasize that proposals can be made by local planners and these are approved if they are structured within established Ministry policy and supported by figures. It was also stressed that the *final* approval of plans rested with authorities of the local government, but to avoid chaos, approval of the central policy-making body is always required.

In addition to funding by the central and local governments, per se, "factory money"—or the profit derived from various industries—is contributed heavily to the support of health services for factory employees.

Differing requirements exist for factories, cities, and for collective farms, so variations of design in function and in size are permitted in the planning of proposed medical facilities, but all personnel policies are set by the Ministry of Health, although each Republic also has its own planning committee and its own Council of Ministers. Each Republic's budget is reviewed annually by the central Ministry in Moscow, and a Republic must justify its need for any anticipated annual increase. The Council of Ministers discusses the submission and suggests allocation of resources. The Supreme Soviet is the final authority of approval.

Our observations confirmed the degree of local autonomy and responsibility in devising health services that had been stressed by the Ministry officials. In talking to many medical administrators, very different ideas were proposed as to how to deliver psychiatric services effectively to patients. For example, although the Vinnitsa area was cited as the best example of the development of psychiatric services in general hospitals and other facilities, in visiting with city officials there, it was apparent that the concept of the specialized mental hospital was still favorably regarded by local authorities.

The Ministry is concerned with, and quite involved in, seeing that enough children are channeled into higher educational programs. In an effort to screen for and search out talent, the Soviets seek to prepare their most promising young people quickly to enter higher educational programs. As the most able emerge, they are selected and sent directly to the medical schools, so that the medical schools will grow in size. The medical schools are independent of universities; substantial clinical space is made available in hospitals for teaching. Branch medical facilities will be established where needed in other republics, through the use of faculty cadres. Standards are established for teaching programs and curricula, but examinations are not developed centrally for use throughout the country. Professors are usually made chairmen of a Commission on Examinations in different schools than their own, however, to help equalize the evaluation of students.

Newly graduated physicians are always assigned to an experienced group, usually in a polyclinic. In accordance with the great emphasis placed by the Russians on the continuing education of their physicians, for each three years in the country and each five years in the city, they are encouraged to take three to five months of postgraduate training. During this additional study, the physician's place is held open for him, and his salary is paid. His medical diploma is only the beginning of a lifetime of learning.

General hospital construction will be expanded to an eventual capacity of 2.5 beds for each 1000 citizens. The Soviets hope to use pilot programs to demonstrate the role of the general hospital in psychiatric care, and they say that they plan to take the next step when it is "educationally correct" to do so. By this they mean that program planners are encouraged to plan psychiatric units in general hospitals, but they are also quite cognizant of the fact that the acceptance of this plan varies widely in Russia.

The Russians stated that at present their psychiatric beds represent 10 to 12 percent of their total hospital beds, whereas in this country, nearly 50 percent of the total number of beds are psychiatric. Furthermore, the Soviets are not "defensive" about the use of psychiatric beds. They put a patient in the bed whenever they think he needs it and hold him as long as they believe necessary.

Although most institutions are actually better staffed than the standard minimum requirement, present staffing standards in Russian psychiatric hospitals (for all shifts) are as follows: In forensic units, there is one psychiatrist for each 25 patients, one registered nurse for 20 patients, and one orderly for every 12 or 13 patients. In acute and disturbed units, one psychiatrist serves 25 patients, one registered nurse serves 30, and one orderly cares for 15 to 20 patients. In sanitaria for children, or general hospital psychiatric units for children, one psychiatrist cares for 25 patients, one registered nurse cares for 30. In quiet wards of nondisturbed patients, there is one psychiatrist and one registered nurse for each 30 patients. Regarding chronic wards, or those that house disturbed patients, there is one psychiatrist for 50 patients, one registered nurse for 40, and one orderly for 20 to 25; in chronic wards for quiet patients, one psychiatrist is assigned for each 80 to 100 patients, one registered nurse is assigned for each 70 patients, and one orderly for each 30 to 35 patients.

In addition, each psychiatric unit has a chief, as well as a chief nurse, an administrative nurse, and a medication nurse. Physical therapists, laboratory workers, and dietitians are provided according to patient load and unit requirements.

This table of organization is eight years old and is undergoing revision to improve staffing ratios. Even now there is a limited flexibility in the table of organization; many institutions have received special approval to add more personnel. Special projects provide justification; for example, workshops and occupational therapy require extra personnel, as do special chemotherapy units, alcoholism programs, postgraduate training and research.

The chief criteria of Russian psychiatric services are availability and accessibility—and this means emergency care at any hour of the night—and specialized diagnostic screening programs in factories, schools and on collective farms. It cannot be emphasized too strongly that the whole concept of the psychiatric hospital is quite different in Russia from that in America. The Russians are much closer to the British belief that psychiatric hospitalization, rather than being quite an abnormal intrusion upon the life experience, is very fre-

quently an understandable part of that experience. To put it as one
Russian psychiatrist did, it seems sometimes very "healthy" for a
person undergoing an emotional crisis to be hospitalized and to
undergo a reconditioning and reconstitution of his defenses against
stress and tension. This philosophy of "normalcy" dominates the attitude of all psychiatric hospital staff. For example, their attitude toward hospital readmissions is so matter-of-fact that it is, at first,
rather shocking to an American visitor. Also, they do not associate
the need for readmission with treatment failure. When it was suggested that, to an American, their rates of readmission seemed high,
they were quick to point out the other side of the coin, namely, that
every readmission had been discharged to the community, and frequently these patients were able to be quite productive before need-
ing readmission for additional shoring up. On the whole, they take a
rather long and philosophical view of the nature of psychiatric illness and they are quite comfortable with the idea that there will
be periods of maladjustments when hospitalization may be the best
protection for the patient.

In another example of the difference in the Russian point of view,
one member of the visiting team of Americans asked a Ministry of
Health official why there was no significant drop in admissions to
inpatient facilities, since so much effort had been put into improving
and intensifying outpatient services. The Ministry official thought
this question an odd one. First of all, he said, improved treatment
services in the dispensaries, factories, the schools and elsewhere, frequently meant that many additional patients with mental illness
who needed hospitalization would be picked up. Secondly, he asked
why the Americans constantly seemed to suggest a rigid dichotomy
between outpatient and inpatient services? Were they not all a part
of the same stream of treatment? And, why did Americans seem to
place a stigma on inpatient treatment?

These differences in the Russian and American approaches to the
handling of mental illness preclude the use of a statistical comparison
to describe the supposed strengths and weaknesses of the two systems.

SUMMARY

Psychiatric care in Russia has been incorporated into their total
medical program, and while the plan has grown and changed through

the years, the basic idea of encompassing all phases of medicine in a fundamental program has been in operation for the past 25 to 30 years. From its inception, the medical program was based on centralized planning which incorporates all phases of medicine, from talent finding, teaching and research, to the clinical practice of its various branches. The operation of this national network of polyclinics and dispensaries, central and regional general hospitals, mental hospitals, sanitaria, special schools for emotionally disturbed, as well as retarded children, is quite impressive. The United States would do well to begin now to plan such a network of integrated programs and services, rather than to constantly decry the shortages and shortcomings that are at least in part the byproduct of our fragmentation of both money and effort. Health care should be made equally available to all and, although we may not choose to support a total health care system similar to that espoused by the Russians, we should be able to harness the creative initiative of a free enterprise system and by some means such as health insurance, provide ready access to quality care for citizens of the United States.

The Russian postgraduate educational system, as it presently exists and as it has been planned for later expansion, gives every promise of being an effective program for keeping the physician up-to-date on current medical knowledge. The goal of quality care seems to underlie a great deal of the medical service in Russia. The missile gap seems to be only one of the gaps which should concern decision-makers in this country. The race to the moon might affect this country's prestige among nations; however, a superb medical care system would certainly put the United States far ahead in any significant race where human values are important.

18

The Mental State of the Norwegian Traitor, Vidkun Quisling

GABRIEL LANGFELDT, M.D.

Professor Emeritus, University of Oslo, Norway

On September 10, 1945, *Eidsivating* court in Oslo condemned the former Norwegian officer, Vidkun Abraham Quisling, to be executed as a traitor. The court had established that before April 9, 1940, Quisling had encouraged the German authorities to attempt a military occupation of Norway. On this date, German military forces invaded Norway at various points in the country. The King and the government left Oslo to escape the Germans, at the same time proclaiming an order of general mobilization. On the same day Quisling broadcast that "the national government," with himself as prime minister, had replaced the former government of Norway. In the same declaration he announced that those who did not obey the new government would be severely punished.

Quisling's court sentence was partly based on the fact that by stating that the Norwegian lawyer, Viggo Hansteen, was engaged in activity dangerous to the country, he had contributed to Hansteen's murder by the Germans. Other offenses were that Quisling refused to support a plea for mercy from 12 Norwegians sentenced to death by the Norwegian Nazi court, with the result that they were all shot, and that Quisling, during the whole occupation and even before, had on several occasions in speeches and articles agitated against the Jews, thus having some responsibility for the transportation of Norwegian Jews to Germany. In addition, Quisling during the occupation had removed from the Royal Palace several pieces of art, silver, and furnishings belonging to the state or to the Royal family.

In the same manner he removed valuables amounting to one million
Norwegian kroner from a society called *Det Norske Selskap* (The
Norwegian Society). From the *frimurerlosjer* (Norwegian Freema-
sons' lodges) he removed valuables worth about 10 million Norwegian
kroner. He was, according to the Norwegian civil penal law, also
sentenced for having appropriated large sums of money for himself
and his ministers. The sentence was appealed to the Supreme Court,
which unanimously condemned him to death. Vidkun Quisling was
shot on October 24, 1945.

Many traits in Quisling and episodes in his life indicate that he
was no ordinary personality. He was a gifted student, especially in
mathematics. But he was lonely and had difficulties in establishing
relationships. He was trained as an officer, but before April 9, 1940,
he was known primarily as secretary to Fridtjof Nansen, who was
helping the Russians and other refugees. Quisling's name was also
known in politics, and he was for a short period the minister of
defense. He later started his own party, *Nasjonal Samling* (National
Coalition).

During the trial, much information concerning Quisling's personality
was given by people who had known him from his college days. Before April 9, 1940, his reputation was excellent among all who knew
him from his youth and also from his work as Nansen's secretary.
During the trial, it was incomprehensible to these people that the
man branded as the prototype of a traitor could be the same helpful
and intellectually gifted person whom they had known.

LEGAL PROCEDURES

Against this background, the usual procedure in Norway for mental
observation is that the chief of police or the state officer request a
preliminary examination of the offender to be carried out by an
expert in forensic psychiatry. He must state whether the offender was
insane at the time of the offense or of the examination, or whether
a doubt exists in this respect. If there is doubt, the expert usually
recommends that the offender undergo a so-called "ordinary" mental examination by two other experts in forensic psychiatry. In the
testimony delivered to the court the experts must also say whether
a state of insanity or unconsciousness exists or existed in the offender
at the time of the offense and whether a condition called "poorly

developed or chronically weakened mental capacities" is present. In addition, the experts must state whether, owing to one of the psychic abnormalities mentioned, there is a risk of relapse. If so, the court is authorized to reduce or withhold punishment and, instead, sentence the offender to a suitable institution of detention for custodial care or treatment.

In Quisling's case two experts were asked on June 8, 1945, to perform a mental examination. On June 18, 1945, they briefly reported that according to the examination Vidkun Quisling was not insane; neither was he suffering from poorly developed or chronically weakened mental capacity. They therefore considered the "ordinary" mental examination to be unnecessary.

When I read these statements in the newspapers, I reacted against them. First, it was not the usual procedure that two experts deliver testimony similar to that given after an "ordinary" mental examination but without the preliminary examination. Second, there was so much curious information in the history of Vidkun Quisling that, in my opinion, an "ordinary" mental observation was absolutely indicated, especially since a death sentence was expected. I contacted the counsel for the defense, Henrik Bergh; however, he would not take the steps necessary to provide an ordinary mental observation. I contacted the chairman of the psychiatric group of the Commission on Forensic Psychiatry in Norway, who stated that the testimony of the experts was preliminary and that the Commission had no obligation to validify it.

EARLY HISTORY

Probably most people in Norway expected, and even demanded, capital punishment for Quisling. Following the execution there were not many comments, and I think people hoped that the tragedy of occupation and the trials following it would be more or less forgotten. However, in recent times, several books and discussions on the personality and actions of Quisling have appeared in Norway. The authors analyzed Quisling predominantly from the historical viewpoint, but they also stressed the curious personality of the traitor. However, none of these authors has a psychiatric background. Many peculiar facets of the personality and actions of Quisling, when analyzed psychiatrically, leave no doubt that he was psychologically abnormal.

By studying the development of his personality and his behavior before and during the German occupation of Norway, as it appears from the descriptions of other authors, from his own literary products, and from the stenographic report of the different trials, I have concluded that Quisling from his younger days was characterized by a tendency to introversion, loneliness, and curious philosophizing. Owing to various disappointments during the years before the German occupation and on the basis of his character anomaly, little by little he evolved as a typical paranoid sociopath with periodic exacerbations of paranoid psychosis.

Vidkun Quisling's father, J. L. Quisling, was a clergyman, described as "a very shy man, preferring to remain in his library with the door closed, and to escape everything but absolutely necessary contact with his congregation." He wrote a most curious book entitled *About the Ghosts and the Angels,* in which he described in detail the bodily and mental characteristics of the angels. Quisling's mother was a melancholic. Vidkun Quisling's brother, Jörgen Quisling, a physician, wrote several peculiar books and was in many ways a deviating personality. In 1931, he published a comprehensive book (1228 pages) entitled *Det Antropokosmiske System (The Anthropocosmic System)* which was characterized by a very strange philosophic ideology similar to that presented in a book by Vidkun Quisling entitled *Universismus.* Jörgen Quisling also published a series of *seksualstudier* (sexual studies), characterized by most curious ideas and a tendency to use new and strange word connections.

DELUSIONS OF GRANDEUR

Vidkun Quisling was looked upon as *primus inter pares* by his school friends. He certainly enjoyed being admired, but was also helpful. However, he is described by all who had known him as a very shut-in personality who had difficulty in communicating. At parties he usually sat alone without speaking.

After the student examination he trained to be an army officer. In this connection it is of interest that from his college days Napoleon was his idol. Perhaps at that time he was already dreaming of playing a role in the development of the world, a need which seems to have steadily increased and which is probably a key to the understanding of his later ideas and mode of behavior. Probably because of his difficulties in relating he seems to have been very introverted, resulting in a tendency to philosophize on obscure matters. In 1929, his book appeared, *About the Matter that Inhabited Worlds Outside Ours and the Significance Caused by It to Our Philosophy of Life.* In this book Quisling maintains that he has succeeded by simple logical reasoning in proving that worlds outside ours exist. He tended to consider as fact what should have been proved, and, like his father and brother, was convinced of the infallibility of his conclusions. The same self-confidence dominated *Universismus* which was probably written during the 1930s. It was never published, and his wife has not allowed anybody to read it. However, a long foreword, much like a summary, was read and recorded during the trial. In essence, Quisling postulates that he has initiated a religion, termed *Universismus,* which explains all problems of life. He purports to be the only thinker who has succeeded in presenting such a religion. He made the following statement regarding this religion: "In this way it will be possible to create an explanation of unity of existence, based on science and experience, which without any doubt gives satisfaction to the claim of the thoughts of men—*Universismus,* the new world religion."

Later in his life several other ideas of grandeur appeared. One of the psychiatric experts, Leikvam, recently stated that after Quisling was imprisoned in 1945, he (Quisling) was convinced that he would have been able to reach the acme in all sections of art and science, except perhaps in the art of painting. Of interest with respect to his paranoid ideas is that during the trial Quisling maintained on several occasions that he believed in a new world of God to come on this earth, and that this faith had been the driving force in all his actions. As to his treachery, he postulated that the occupation was a trial by ordeal and that the love of his country was the motivating force for his action. In spite of the fact that as prime minister during the German occupation he had approved the death sentence of many Norwegians and had agitated against the Jews and against Norwegian clergymen and teachers, he steadily maintained that he had only been helpful to his countrymen. In his defense he identified himself with St. Olav of Norway. After he received the death sentence, he wrote in a letter to his brother, "Well, now I am going to die as a martyr, like Jesus Christ." His counsel for the defense and Leikvam steadily maintained that Quisling had acted in good faith during the whole occupation.

Curiously, in 1939 Quisling, quite privately, drew up a detailed proposal for peace which he sent to the governments of France, Britain, and Germany. It should also be mentioned that at the end of the occupation when it was quite evident that the Germans would lose the war, Quisling arranged that his church department accept his wish to be appointed a clergyman in his home community. As motivation for accepting the application, a publication from the department explained that it was the wish of the prime minister to continue his influence on the development of the world according to his religious philosophy. This application was stressed by the counsel for the defense as one of the curious traits in Quisling's personality, demonstrating, as he expressed it, that "there must in the defendant be something physical or psychic, which none of us, nor the medical doctors, understand." During the trial it was evident to everybody that Quisling, with the purpose of maintaining the illusion of his reverent personality, made use of lies, falsifications of memory, and repressions in a systematic manner which—in my experience—is only encountered in paranoid personalities.

To understand the development of Quisling's paranoid disorder it must be mentioned that in 1923 he had applied to the military authorities for permission to continue his work with Nansen for the refugees but was refused. This left him very disappointed, and he became even more lonely and bitter. However, he continued to display an overwhelming need to play an important role in world affairs. Despite the fact that his involvement with Russia had been unsuccessful, he stated that, "I was the one who performed the work in Russia; this is something I say to no disparagement of Nansen." It is noteworthy that during 1924 to 1926 he made an attempt to contact six Communist party leaders and workers to offer them his services, which were not accepted.

Later on, he tried to play a role in Norwegian politics, and succeeded in being elected to the cabinet in a farmer party government. However, he encountered much opposition, especially from the workers' party. Enthusiastic as he was about the leadership principle, it is not surprising that the idea of Nazism engaged him from the beginning of the thirties, resulting in his organization on May 12, 1933, of the Norwegian Nazi party (*Nasjonal Samling*).

SUMMARY

Vidkun Quisling belonged to a family of which two members—his father and his brother—had a tendency toward strange philosophic speculations. From early school years Quisling appeared to be gifted, but introverted and lonely. He also tended toward philosophic speculations and wrote two books, one of which postulated a new religion. The need to play a crucial role in the development of the world became a dominant trait, which was closely associated with his religious beliefs. Gradually, he became completely blinded by his mission in the world situation. In addition to his grandiose ideas in the religious sphere, he also displayed ideas of grandeur in his proposition for peace between the nations at war in 1939. Even after the Germans had lost the war, he hoped to continue to influence development in Norway "and further on" by election as a clergyman. A dominant characteristic of Quisling's was the steadily increasing lack of insight into himself as well as his tendency to suppress facts and falsify memories.

In my opinion, Quisling showed a typical picture of paranoia with ideas of grandeur and of being a prophet. The many abnormal traits in his character and history should have spurred the psychiatric experts to recommend that he be subjected to an "ordinary" mental observation, which was the usual procedure in such trials in Norway. Although this might not have saved his life—public opinion was felt to have influenced the verdict very strongly—the usual humanitarian and legal procedures should have been carried out, and I feel that it was deplorable that this was not done.

19

The Psychosocial Effect of the Eichmann Trial on Israeli Society

JULIUS ZELLERMAYER, M.D.

Professor and Chairman of Psychiatry
Hadassah University Hospital, Jerusalem, Israel

The Eichmann trial was a very significant chapter in Israeli history. It occurred at a time of avoidance from public discussion of the subject of the catastrophe and the annihilation of six million Jews. Most people in Israel before and after the establishment of the State in 1948 refused somehow to feel the full impact of what had happened in the death-factories of Nazi Germany. The struggle for independence and statehood absorbed them to such a degree and necessitated such a mobilization of fighting spirit that to identify with that part of the nation that had demonstrated its defenselessness was at that time nearly impossible. There could be no identification with those who had perished. On all levels in schools during the period 1950 to 1960 the shameful events were circumvented. Israelis born after the Second World War drew a sharp line of division between themselves and those who had become victims of Nazi barbarism. A deep schism threatened national and historic consciousness. Continuity of history was on the verge of breaking down. At a time when, with the establishment of the State of Israel, a strong need for identity and solidarity was of utmost importance, the self-image of the nation was threatened by the confrontation with its immediate painful and shameful past.

This state of affairs was reversed nearly overnight by the Eichmann trial. The shame, disgust, and contempt felt before about passively suffered extermination disappeared, as it became known that resistance had been fierce and heroic, and that, where it was weak or absent, it had been smashed to pieces by a new system of dehumanization, planned and executed by a monstrous machine to which humans with normal resistances could not easily stand up. That this same power had overrun a whole continent and subdued it to its wishes, and that millions of others were likewise exterminated, although they had at their disposal the protection of their own states and armies, had the deep effect of restoration of national pride. The trial thus corrected dangerous, distorted perceptions and misinterpretations. The most intensive revival of horrifying memories, the reenactment of the catastrophe, but this under the completely changed historic conditions of the new sovereign state, had a remarkable, cathartic effect. By combining shame with pride and anger with triumph, historic continuity and national identity were reestablished.

If before the trial, doubts were expressed about the undesirable effect the trial might have on the population as a whole and on various of its subgroups—children, youth, survivors, and others—after the trial, opinion was unanimous that the trial was a major event, not so much and not alone in its legal or historic dimensions but in its psychosocial implications. The fragmented society of the Israel population composed in 1961, at the start of the trial, of about 37 percent Israel born, 26 percent immigrants from Oriental countries, and 35 percent immigrants from European countries, about 60 percent of whom had arrived after the establishment of the State, now realized its common fate. In May and June, 1967, when once again it was threatened with extermination, the lesson of the trial stood its historic test.

This certainly is a schematization. Naturally, the reaction of the Israel born, the orientals, the old European immigrants, and the survivor group were different from each other. A few basic attitudes, though, were shared by most of them, of which I would mention a deep conscious guilt about not having done enough to save relatives and friends, and a sense of utter perplexity about the indifference of the civilized world to the fate of a defenseless people.

To learn that governments and churches of the western world did practically nothing to prevent the massacre, and this even after El-Alamein and Stalingrad, at which time two million were known to have been gassed in the death factories, but another four million could still have been saved, was a most shocking revelation. This revelation could not but create distrust against the world at large, which was not fully overcome until now.

Let me turn now to some of the various subgroups. The survivor group itself may be divided into those coming directly from the concentration and extermination camps, numbering each 80,000 and about 300,000 others—active partisans, underground fighters, and those who had lived with false Aryan papers. Most had accomplished a moderate psychosocial adaptation after their arrival in the new homeland. They had married, borne children, and adjusted, at least superficially, to society and work. Yet beneath their performance level one could often find that they were guilt ridden because of their sheer survival in the face of the massive losses of their next of kin. They were in a state of chronic nonclinical depression, reluctant to communicate their traumatic experiences, suspicious of the Israeli environment, suffering from various somatic ailments, usually diagnosed as vegetative dystonias, for which they avoided application for psychiatric help. They were fixated in their memory of oppression and death, from which they suffered but which they did not attempt to give up. In more extreme cases they manifested passivity and apathy, interrupted only at times by outbursts of anger against others and themselves. Isolated in their emotional shell, they could not share their memories, guilts, and shames with anybody, including physicians. It was beyond their capacity to describe verbally their unique experiences, and it was equally impossible for the listener to fully comprehend the words and tales that he heard from the survivor. In this respect, the trial was extremely effective. What they themselves could not verbalize, was now verbalized for them by the prosecution, the witnesses, reporters, and the press. Their uncommunicable experiences were now conceptualized, their humiliations explained, their inability to resist excused, their guilt about their survival resolved. Parents who until then could not talk with their children born in Israel about their own experiences in the concentration camps, who had covered up nearly every detail of their own former history and that of their extinguished family, now for the first time could tell their children what had happened, and face them as individuals with a personal and a family history of their own. Children learned in this way for the first time about grandparents, uncles and aunts, and about places that until then were kept deliberately and systematically from their knowledge.

An even stranger effect was that some of the survivors, who until then had refused to claim restitution from the German authorities because of shame and guilt for having survived, permitted themselves now to demand compensation from the hated persecutor, with whom, until then, they had refused to have dealings of any kind. Their delay in lodging their claims beyond the legal deadline made them suspect to the authorities, both in Israel and Germany. In more than one situation it was necessary to explain to the authorities the specific psychologic constellation that had contributed to the late application for their restitution claims. The subsequent compensation was followed in many instances by reactive depressive moods.

The trial had another effect. Most of the survivor patients were not motivated and not accessible to psychotherapy. They resisted remembering and reexperiencing the psychotraumatic experiences and refused to be helped and restored to the pleasures of living. In addition, the psychotherapists were part of that other world with whom they could hardly establish rapport, whom they perceived as lacking in sensitivity, and to whom they related with distrust. It cannot be denied that the attitude of the psychotherapists themselves was not encouraging. Many of them shared the reserved or even negative attitudes of the public at large in regard to the survivors. Most of them were preholocaust Europeans. They, too, felt guilt because they had survived, while other members of their family or close friends had perished. These guilt feelings were transformed into unspoken accusations against the survivors, and as long as these prevailed, psychotherapeutic constructive empathy could not be established.

The psychosocial drama of the trial changed this situation. Some of the survivors dared psychotherapeutic exploration, some of the psychotherapists felt the need and the ability to extend their skills. On the whole not too much could be achieved, as the psychopathologies were of a progressive chronicity and only superficially accessible. The changed social and family situation after the trial had, for some, a positive effect. Had we better understood and been better emotionally prepared to deal with the survivors earlier, some irreparable deterioration could perhaps have been prevented.

Until 1959 to 1960 Israeli psychiatrists had some blind spots in respect to the specific traumatization of Nazi atrocities and the resulting psychopathologic effects. When called upon to give expert evaluation of the psychiatric consequences of persecution and oppression, psychiatrists in Israel, as elsewhere, tended to assess these disorders in terms of those concepts that were relevant in regard to post-traumatic conditions of war or civilian casualties. Only in the late 1950s, and especially under the influence of the publications of Venzlaff, Kolle, Strauss, Baeyer, and others, did a new approach to these postoppressive clinical conditions develop. Again, we must regret it, but had all of us begun to understand sooner, unjustified disadvantageous psychiatric expert opinion could have been avoided.

On the other hand it must be mentioned that for many, survivors and others, participation in the public trial was beyond their capacity. They could not listen to the radio nor read the papers, and they persisted in excluding from their awareness anything relating to the catastrophe. Some of the postconcentration camp patients withdrew even more during the trial. Some experienced strong persecutory anxieties and dissociative states. Fortunately, these exacerbations subsided after days or weeks. The same happened to some Europeans who had immigrated into Palestine before 1939. Strong guilt feelings had appeared about those they had failed to rescue. Anxieties and depressions of transitory character turned them for a time to psychiatric help, which in most instances improved their condition rapidly.

It may perhaps be interesting to know that, for some, the trial meant the closing of a chapter. Justice was done. The criminal was executed. Israel had taken its revenge. One could now turn one's back on the cruel and haunting past and gradually resume contact with the world and even with post-Nazi Germany. This readiness to draw a line between past and present, between bad and good Germans, was strongly resented by the great majority.

This is a rough schematization. Not all survivors were clinically depressed, apathetic, etc. Not all psychiatrists failed to understand and help. Many survivors made good adjustments, especially those of the active partisans and those who belonged to the skilled and academic socioeconomic groups. There were other differences: Those of the 30- to 40-year age group during the oppression adjusted better than the younger ones, but behind the facade of normality of most of these, the scars of their oppressive experiences could be detected, although in these instances mostly the attempt to keep a normal facade was an extremely strong defense mechanism; to officers and regular soldiers, in which not alone the Eichmann trial and all it revealed were brought to their attention, but also the magnificent heroism of those of the Gentile world, who were presented as the "Righteous and the Just," as the representatives of human dignity and the moral spirit unconquerable even under the most adverse conditions. This balancing operation was not a strategic maneuver. It originated in a genuine feeling that refused to conceive the whole world in the image of Eichmann, Hitler, and the Nazi system as a whole. A special institution was founded by the State to honor the moral heroes among the Gentiles of all nations. Approximately 400 have been granted special honorary awards in a much publicized ceremony, and many more will be honored in the future, promoting reconciliation between Jews and Gentiles.

But even more significant were the adaptational devices destined to channel the mourning process of the nation as a whole. At the belated stage of the Eichmann trial, when confronted collectively with the holocaust, comparable in its uniqueness only to what happened 2000 years ago with the destruction of the Temple and the loss of national independence, one could not rely on spontaneous recovery alone. Planned social action had to be instituted.

In terms of individual psychology, depression, guilt, and intense selfdeprecation follow loss of objects. But what is the meaning of six million lost? Can one fully grasp such an event, or does it exceed our normal mental and psychic capacity? Is it more or less painful in terms of object loss, and what are the psychologic reactions of the individual, the group or society at large in such a situation? Do individuals react differently, when sharing the grief with others, their whole nation, and when their loss has lost its individual character and has become a national catastrophe? Does depression become collective, is guilt transformed into something else and, furthermore, do all these otherwise regular reactions develop, when the threat of extermination has to be faced permanently as in the case of Israel, whose neighbors declare openly that they intend to finish the job left over by the Nazis? These are open sociopsychologic problems.

In terms of social action and in order to cope with such an unusual event, an interesting plan was initiated. The mass of six million was translated into 16,000 annihilated Jewish communities, which could more easily be grasped and then commemorated in a more meaningful and concrete manner. Accordingly, a reconstructive scheme was devised by which schools and classes began to adopt, the way parents do with children, destroyed Jewish communities. School

classes, with the help of their teachers and educators, decided on an
identification process with one specific lost community by way of
studying its history, geography, culture, its leading personalities, and
especially the vicissitudes of that community in the last decades up
to the extermination, becoming through this learning and identification process heirs and perpetuators of those who had perished. This
movement of adopting communities has, during the years after the
Eichmann trial, gained in momentum. It has encompassed schools
of the various ethnic groups and has thus become not alone a living
bridge from the past to the present but an integrating force, establishing cross identification of children and youngsters from Oriental
communities with those of central Europe. Nearly 500 communities
have been adopted. One can assume this will have far-reaching socio-
therapeutic implications. In a world facing many man-made disasters
and societal dilemmas of ethnocentricisms and segregations, this psychosocial experiment may serve as a model to be applied elsewhere.

The problem of how to teach this subject matter in schools remains
unsettled. Until now an authoritative textbook of the history of the
holocaust has not been produced. Two educational tendencies oppose
each other: the one attempting primarily to preserve the memory
for future generations, the other to study and learn it, objectively,
and scientifically. Lately, the second tendency is becoming more
pronounced and widespread. It is maintained that to study what
happened by way of critical analysis must not be offensive to the
victims and that the 20 years passed since the catastrophe enable
and oblige the use of objective criteria and evaluations. A meaningful
learning situation can be developed now for another reason. As is
well known, Israeli youth is soberly realistic. For good or for worse
it has adopted a pattern of nonemotionality as a result of the unin-
terrupted struggle for national survival and the unavoidable sacri-
fices this entails. They know that the subject matter of the catastrophe must be assimilated by them although it cannot be easily
handled according to this pattern of nonemotionality. The exposure
to the facts of the holocaust coincided with that phase of their own
development, when aggressive impulses play a major role in their
own lives. Their age-determined natural tendency would motivate
them to identify with the aggressor; their unavoidable identification
with the victim prohibits such an outcome. Fortunately, this impasse
can now be handled more easily, because one emotional obstacle, to
become exposed to the catastrophe period and its conflictive impact,

has receded into the background. The success of establishing a state, of fighting successfully, has restored their self-esteem. They need not anymore feel shame and disgust, as they have ample proof of their invincible spirit. Whatever befell a former generation, they can now attempt to understand without identificatory anxieties. They do now identify with heroes of their present and past but are mature enough to feel that it is not heroism for its own sake, but in the service of their existence and survival that it is demanded of them. It is with this new realism that they approach the subject matter of the holocaust. They wish to understand by way of a critical analysis the roots of antisemitism, the degeneration of it into geno-cide, the part played by the Jews themselves in their extermination, the shortcomings of the leadership, and the factors that made them blind to their impending disasters. Since the trial of Eichmann this preparedness to learn has widened and deepened. New data could be introduced into the curricula, as both the Hebrew University Department of General and of Jewish Contemporary History, as well as the research divisions of the Institute for the Remembrance of the Holocaust (Jad Kashe) through their more recent contributions could throw additional light on many, until now, hidden topics. The fact, too, that the teachers themselves are now mostly Israelis with-out the kind of personal involvement that characterized those who were themselves survivors of the holocaust, is promoting a more real-istic learning situation. But in this respect we are only in the first phase of this development.

The entire range of problems posed by Eichmann as a person and a case is beyond the scope of this review. It was the first time that the Israeli public sat face to face with the robot murderer, the bureaucrat of destruction. It was for everyone a bewildering experi-ence. In our present context, however, what is relevant is not how he really was as a clinical psychiatric patient, but rather how he was perceived and understood by the public and some of its subgroups.

The intention of the prosecution was clearly to present him as one of the major criminals, not as a subordinate to his superiors, whose commands he had to carry out. It is doubtful whether this objective was fully achieved. The independent part that he had played in the monstrous extermination was proved in the trial beyond any doubt, and there were no doubts about his guilt in the legal sense, but most people could not really make up their minds how to classify him. It was felt by many, those in direct contact with him and those observing him from some distance, that he was a weakling—in terms of personality, a nonentity. Feelings towards him were less of genuine hatred and more of disgust and contempt. But this did not obscure the issue for anyone; just the contrary. Hitlers do not realize their demonic designs in a human vacuum. Totalitarian systems function through Eichmann's and his ilk and though they may be mediocrities or banalities in the sense of Hannah Arendt, in the hands of a totalitarian bureaucracy they become instrumental for the killing of millions. As the Israeli intellectual community learned more about him and his socio-political context, the interdependence of social structure and personality type posed itself, for them, as the real problem. In various publications much concern was expressed about these aspects. The moral responsibility of the individual, the clash between law and conscience, the moral grounds and obligation to disobey immoral orders of the state authority were dealt with by various authors. Some wondered whether the undue emphasis in our psychologic theory and education practice on the socialization process in the formative years of development may not contribute to undesirable conformity to the group and prepare, thereby, the ground for later authoritarianism, if it is not balanced early by internalization of nongroup-determined moral standards. Moral autonomy as well as individuation, the first especially a much neglected problem in psychology, were given renewed consideration and significance as those psychic counterforces destined to better resist the immoralities and insanities of the mass state. That knowledge of the processes and laws that govern the formation of these psychic structures is at the moment insufficient was seriously regretted and, especially, that as long as this gap in our knowledge exists, education in this area remains without scientific orientation.

This is a sketchy report. Only few aspects could be selected for presentation. Israel is a new-old nation. Three thousand years of history are at the same time a blessing and a burden.

It is no wonder that at this phase of the reestablished State in the old homeland the search for identity is rather acute. The effects of the trial on some of the population, both in its positive and negative aspects, were actually only side effects. The real significance was the confrontation of the nation with itself, with the Gentile world, the threats to its existence, and the lessons to be learned. Future historians and social scientists will be able to assess the place it holds in the process of national self-definition.

20

The Psychiatrist's Power in Civil Commitment: A Knife That Cuts Both Ways

A. M. DERSHOWITZ

Professor of Criminal Law
Harvard University School of Law

An important, if subtle, consequence of psychiatric involvement in the legal process has been the gradual introduction of a medical model in the place of the law's efforts to articulate legally relevant criteria. This may be illustrated by reference to the process known as civil commitment of the mentally ill, whereby almost one million persons are today confined behind the locked doors of state mental hospitals, though never convicted of a crime.

The criteria for confinement are so vague that courts sit—when they sit at all—merely to review decisions made by psychiatrists. Indeed, the typical criteria—mental illness, need of treatment, likely to harm self or others—are so meaningless as even to preclude effective review. And this will continue, so long as the law continues to ask the dispositive questions in medical rather than legal functional terms because the medical model does not ask the proper questions, or asks them in meaningless vague terms: Is the person mentally ill? Is he dangerous to himself or to others or in need of care or treatment?

Nor is this the only way to ask questions to which the civil commitment process is responsive. It will be instructive to restate the problem of civil commitment without employing medical terms and to see whether the answers suggested differ from those now given.

There are, in every society, people who may cause trouble if not confined. The trouble may be serious (such as homicide); trival (making offensive remarks); or somewhere in between (forging checks). The trouble may be directed at others, at the person himself, or at both. It may be very likely that he will cause trouble, or fairly likely, or fairly unlikely. In some instances this likelihood may be considerably reduced by a relatively short period of involuntary confinement; in others, a longer period may be required with no assurances of reduced risk; while in still others, the likelihood can never be significantly reduced. Some people will have fairly good insight into the risks they pose; others will have poor insight.

What sorts of anticipated harm warrant involuntary confinement? How likely must it be that the harm will occur? Must there be a significant component of harm to others, or may it be to self alone? If harm to self is sufficient, must the person also be incapable, because he lacks insight, of weighing the risks to himself against the costs of confinement? How long a period of involuntary confinement is justified to prevent which sorts of harms? Must the likelihood of the harm increase as its severity decreases or as the component of harm to others decreases?

These questions are complex, but this is as it should be, for the business of balancing the liberty of the individual against the risks a free society must tolerate is very complex. That is the business of the law, and these are the questions which need asking and answering before liberty is denied. Nor have I simply manufactured these questions. They are the very questions which are being implicitly answered every day by psychiatrists, but they are not being openly asked, and many psychiatrists do not realize that they are, in fact, answering them.

The initial and fundamental question which must be asked by any system authorizing incarceration is which harms are sufficiently serious to justify to this rather severe sanction? This question is asked and answered in the criminal law by the substantive definitions of crime. Thus, homicide is a harm which justifies the sanction of imprisonment; miscegenation does not; and adultery is a close case about which reasonable people may, and do, disagree. It is difficult to conceive of a criminal process which does not make some effort at articulating these distinctions. Imagine, for example, a penal code which simply makes it an imprisonable crime to cause injury to self or others, without defining injury; or a penal code which authorizes incarceration for anyone who performs an act regarded as injurious by a designated expert, such as a psychiatrist or penologist.

Yet, this is precisely the situation that prevails with civil commitment. The statutes authorize preventive incarceration of mentally ill persons who are likely to injure themselves or others. Generally, "injure" is not further defined in the statutes or in the case law, and the critical decision—whether a predicted pattern of behavior is sufficiently injurious to warrant incarceration—is relegated to the psychiatrist's unarticulated judgments.

Some psychiatrists are perfectly willing to provide their own personal opinions—often falsely disguised as expert opinions—about which harms are sufficiently serious. But as one would expect, some psychiatrists are political conservatives while others are liberals; some place a greater premium on safety, others on liberty. Their opinions about which harms do and which do not justify confinement probably cover the range of opinions one would expect to encounter in any educated segment of the public. But they are opinions about matters which each of us is as qualified to form as they are. Thus, this most fundamental decision is almost never made by the legislature or the courts. Often it is never explicitly made by anybody, and when it is explicitly made, it is by an unelected and unappointed expert operating outside the area of his expertise.

There is another important question which rarely gets asked in the civil commitment process. How likely should the predicted event have to be to justify preventive incarceration? Not only do psychiatrists determine the degree of likelihood which should be required for incarceration, they also decide whether that degree of likelihood exists in any particular case.

But just how expert are psychiatrists in making the sort of predictions upon which incarceration is presently based? Considering the heavy, indeed exclusive, reliance the law places on psychiatric predictions, one would expect there to be numerous follow-up studies establishing their accuracy. Over this past year, with the help of two researchers, I conducted a thorough survey of all the published literature on the prediction of antisocial conduct. We read and summarized many hundreds of articles, monographs, and books. Surprisingly, we were able to discover fewer than a dozen studies which followed up psychiatric predictions of antisocial conduct. And even more surprising, these few studies strongly suggest that psychiatrists are even less accurate when compared with other professionals such as pychologists, social workers, and correctional officials, and also when compared to actuarial devices, such as prediction or experience tables. Even more significant for legal purposes, it seems that psychiatrists are particularly prone to one type of error—over-prediction. They tend to predict antisocial conduct in many instances where it would not, in fact, occur.

One reason for this prediction is that a psychiatrist almost never learns about his erroneous predictions of violence, for predicted assailants are generally incarcerated and have little opportunity to prove or disprove the prediction; but he always learns about his erroneous predictions of non-violence, often from newspaper headlines announcing the crime. This higher visibility of erroneous predictions of non-violence inclines him, whether consciously or unconsciously, to overpredict violent behavior.

The lesson of this experience is that no legal rule should ever be phrased in medical terms; that no legal decision should ever be turned over to psychiatrists. And civil commitment of the mentally ill is a legal problem; whenever compulsion is used or freedom denied— whether by the state, the church, the union, the university, or the psychiatrist—the issue becomes a legal one and lawyers must quickly become involved.

21

Notes on Charisma

JOHN M. CALDWELL, M.D.

Formerly, Professor and Chairman of Psychiatry
University of Miami School of Medicine

Charisma is a word that has become extremely popular in the last several months; this popularity may be deserved, but the usage has varied widely.

Howard Rome, in an unpublished paper, "The Expanding Domain of Psychiatric Competence," writes of the charisma of psychiatry. Others refer to persons as charismatic, and an advertisement extolling the virtues of a new perfume called "Charisma" proclaims, "The woman who wears it, has it."

In a recent paper, also unpublished, entitled "The Nature and Nurture of Charisma," Raymond Headlee summarizes his interests in, and concepts of, charisma. He defines it as "the interplay between those who seek quasi-divine power and those who seem to seek others who have this personal mystique."

John L. Lewis is perhaps the first person in modern times to whom the term was applied. It is reported that "charisma" was used by Daniel Bell in an article on Lewis published in *Fortune Magazine* 21 years ago.

Since then lists have been compiled of persons having charisma as well as lists of those who do not. Included among those who allegedly have charisma may be Charles de Gaulle, Ronald Reagan, William Buckley, Moshe Dayan, the late Martin Luther King, and all members of the Kennedy family. Among those who perhaps are not overly endowed with charisma are Lester Maddox, Alexei Kosygin, George Meany, and Shirley Temple Black.

"Charis" was, in the Iliad, the wife of Hepaestus. Later, the name applied to any one of the three Graces or "charities," reflecting fertility, charm, and beauty in general.

In Webster's New International Dictionary, charis is defined somewhat as follows:

> A special divine or spiritual gift; a special divine endowment conferred upon a believer as an evidence of the experience of divine grace, and fitting him for the life, work, or office to which he was called; a grace, as a miraculously given power of healing or of speaking with tongues, or of prophesying, etc., attributed to some of the early Christians.

The Oxford English Dictionary, in its 13 Volume Edition, has the following to say:

> *Charism*: A free gift or favour specially vouchsafed by God; a grace, a talent . . . miraculous gift of healing. The gift of prophecy was that charism which enabled its possessors to utter, with the authority of inspiration, divine strains of warning.

In his paper, Headlee states that the charismatic person is usually power-oriented rather than esthetically, socially, economically, religiously, or theoretically oriented. The different forms of power include assertive power, e.g., Huey Long; creative power, e.g., Franz Alexander or Freud; or factual power, e.g., Alexander Hamilton. Charisma emerges as assertive power with the charismatic person having absolute knowledge and the ability to manipulate a group for predetermined goals. Enhancing the quality of charisma may be such attributes as a distinctive physical appearance, social grace, political presence, high energy output, and calmness of demeanor. Included among the dangers of possessing charisma are physical exhaustion, withdrawal, homoerotic behavior, depression, and paranoid states.

Certain conditions contribute to the nurture of charisma, according to Headlee. Once a position of being a charismatic person is established, it tends to continue in spite of negative or positive judgments on the part of others. The charismatic person is basically noninvolved emotionally with followers and covers this attitude with a pseudo-humanistic facade. One cannot be a leader without some followers, so there is then the task of recruiting of both active and passive followers. The charismatic leader characteristically promotes humility and self-abasement, e.g., the cult of the antiself. The interlocking relationship with followers may be on the basis of hatred, power, sex, aggression, or love.

There are few papers on charisma to be found in the literature, but there is an interesting discussion of charismatic leadership by George Devereux in Volume IV of *Psychoanalysis and the Social Sciences*. Devereux feels that charismatic leadership is one not socially justified but is derived from an external agency with which the leader is felt to entertain a closer relationship than other persons do. Sometimes this agency is "the people"—at other times, the leader, is the true interpreter of some doctrine. Charismatic leaders may, in the course of time, accede to some status or office.

The charismatic leader is a latter-day representative of the parental figure, as the child sees the parent during the stage of delegated omnipotence. Such infantile conceptions of the adult role are not automatically outgrown when the subject himself reaches at least chronologic maturity.

There are, perhaps, two types of fantasies about "instinctual paradise." One is the "Garden of Eden" or "Golden Age" fantasy involving the past, i.e., infantile bliss. The other is the "Utopian" fantasy involving the future, i.e., adult pleasures. The psychopath does not behave like a child but tries hard to act grown up. He does so, however, by conforming not to real standards of mature behavior, but to infantile ideas about what constitutes adult conduct. He behaves as he thinks his parents once behaved. It is Devereux' thesis that in a crisis, as defined above, people regress to a state of delegated omnipotence, and, in accordance with the ideology of that developmental state, demand a leader who conforms to infantile ideas of adult behavior. This may explain why society-in-crisis selects so many psychopaths in the role of charismatic leader.

Similarly, Toynbee, in *A Study of History*, wrote that during a breakdown of civilizations certain trends may appear in, or be advocated by, leaders as forms of escape. These forms may be futurism or archaism, withdrawal and return, detachment and transfiguration. The charismatic leader may advocate or participate in such fundamental trends.

It would seem that institutions could be considered charismatic wherein such qualities are to be found as healing, inspiration, graces, or talents. Individuals having charismatic qualities may employ them in the service of others, and there August Aichorn, Father Flanagan of Boy's Town, and men like them come to mind. Some of our own psychiatric fraternity, such as the psychiatric dynasties of Walter Freeman, might be considered as having charisma. While on one hand, certain political figures are humanistically oriented, others are exploitively oriented. This opposite side of the coin could be represented, as well, by such confidence men as Ponzi or Kreuger, who perhaps had some charismatic attributes.

It would seem to the author that from available information and sources cited charisma involves (to a greater or lesser degree) certain qualities or conditions, such as the following:

1. A religious theme.

2. An empathic understanding of the needs of others by the leader and a promise of fulfillment.

3. An altruistic facade, real or assumed, with the ingredient of "non-self" or Sainthood," or both.

4. An ego-regression by followers, with the expression of primitive urges permitted, the child-parent relationship fostered, and a substitutive super-ego provided.

The author recalls a few persons who might be considered as having charismatic qualities. One was the leader of a boys' camp in California during the early 1950s. A visit was made to the camp to meet with the leader in order to find out something about the factors that had led to the camp's reputation and success in rehabilitating delinquent boys. Interest in the matter had been stimulated by success reported of a school in England in a book entitled *Mr. Lywood's Answer* by Michael Burn. On a personal visit to the camp, it was discovered that the leader had died a month previously. A grieving staff was in the process of dismantling the rustic buildings and discontinuing the program. Upon inquiry as to what the leader had been like as a person, the statement was made, "If ever Jesus Christ had been reincarnated on earth, this man was that reincarnation." Shades of August Aichorn!

While no attempt will be made to evaluate Harry Stack Sullivan's contribution to psychiatry, there is little doubt that he was a magnetic person and attracted many followers. It was noted by the author that a number of individuals in Washington emulated Sullivan in dress, manner, selection of phrases, and similar doctor-patient relationships, including the time and spacing of appointments. In a supervisory seminar it is remembered that Sullivan spoke to a woman student, who was reporting on her patient, in the following terms, "You remind me of a phlegmatic cow leaping from mountain peak to mountain peak. I have no idea how you get from one place to another. Suppose you descend into the valley and tell me how you are traveling from one point to another." The author asked his supervisor about Sullivan's apparent caustic approach and was told that he, the supervisor, had used some of Sullivan's phrases to patients and had promptly lost every one of them. Sullivan had an empathic understanding of his patients and could say things that on the surface would seem to antagonize, but in reality would do nothing of the sort. Any imitator, however, was likely to meet with disaster. While there was, perhaps, no religious theme, Sullivan undoubtedly had an empathic understanding of the needs of others, both peers and patients. He operated largely in an altruistic setting, and a substitutive super-ego was provided. The criteria for the use of the word charisma as applied to Sullivan are considered to have been established.

Another individual who possessed outstanding qualities of leadership was William Menninger. In his life there was a strong religious theme and his dedication to the welfare of others was a, if not the, dominant theme in his own life. He chose psychiatry as the means of achieving his goals. It would be presumptuous to say what his goals were, but a certain latitude may be allowed the author by reason of a close, though intermittent, relationship over a period of some two decades. Again, no attempt will be made to evaluate the very substantial contribution that Bill Menninger made to psychiatry and to the American scene. His impact on individuals, while subtle, was almost universally effective in obtaining support for his goals. These goals seemed to be directed toward bringing about a better way of life for all men, and toward the removal of obstacles in the way of achieving that better life here on earth. His characteristic phrase was "Did you do good today?"—the "good" meaning did you do something to improve the possibility of a better way of living for others. If "good" could not be reported, one met, nevertheless, with an optimistic attitude—if not today, tomorrow. In short summary, Bill Menninger's life was characterized by religious themes and empathic understanding of human needs, a truly altruistic way of living, and

the encouragement and support of others to "do good" and to mini-
mize that which was interfering, impeding, or undesirable.

The individuals mentioned above might be considered as exempli-
fying positive charisma. Less is known of individuals employing
charismatic attributes in a negative or destructive manner. There
are examples, however, and hopefully a report of psychiatric studies
in the future will be made.

Section III

ADMINISTRATION AND SERVICES

.

22

The Public Mental Hospital in Modern Psychiatry: What Everyone Knows or Ought To

FRANCIS J. O'NEILL, M.D.

Director, Central Islip State Hospital, New York;
Clinical Professor of Psychology, New York School of Psychiatry

---

"It is a fact," said Thomas W. Salmon 35 years ago, "that every stage (including community health programs) in the long and painful history of the care of the insane from 1247, when the first institution for the insane in England was provided, could actually be witnessed in some American community this afternoon" (1).

In a society where change is often misinterpreted as progress and the value of an effort is equated with its cost, there is a tendency to give traditional methods which have functioned effectively despite highly restrictive economic limitations, crippling political expediencies, and neglect by urban psychiatry and the public less than their due.

The public mental hospital, the core of psychiatric treatment in America for the past 100 years, is now undergoing a revolution in terms of its orientation, its goals, and its opportunities. Under the impetus of an increasing general awareness of mental illness, which includes the role and structure of the public mental hospital, there has been a tendency to emphasize the negative aspects of these institutions and to de-emphasize their value. An image of the public mental hospital consisting of forbidding buildings, untrained staff, and an inadequate number of professionals—all contributing to the illness of patients by encouraging chronicity—is now current. That these institutions have been effectively serving their populations in terms of good treatment and quick discharge of those who respond has been given less than fair expression. Consequently, the efforts of mental health workers struggling against odds in our public institutions are being undetermined and disorted.

PERIOD OF CHANGE

We are now witnessing in the mental health field a period of radical and massive change. Public mental hospitals are considered by many to be too large and impersonal. There are many people who feel that large institutions should be fractionated into smaller, more personalized units. Some feel that public mental hospitals should be completely abolished, although this view is likely to be held by those without personal experience of a severely disturbed person in the home; the trauma invoked by such a situation is often so disintegrating that removal of the severely disturbed patient from the home is the only way to avoid the possibility of additional psychiatric disturbances developing in the immediate family.

There is a growing emphasis on community involvement and primary prevention, almost to the exclusion of existing programs. New and expensive organizations and programs are being created along with unique professional and nonprofessional roles. Theoretic foci are being broadened so that various health-related disciplines that attempt to encompass the full range of problems of man in society are developing. Such lofty aims are laudable and excite the imagination of the public. A broad clinical-personal-social interactional approach is emerging. As a result, drastic innovations in organizational structure, program development, clinical practice and training, and the utilization of para-medical personnel in areas often beyond their expertise are being carried out and implemented with a very limited theoretic base. With today's compelling need for change and a general impatience with the status quo, we have pushed ahead without making a major effort in intellectual enterprise, i.e., in theory construction, research, teaching, and pilot programs and evaluations. The result has been general chaos and prodigious expenditures, with insufficient attention to the development of a systematic convergence of scientific, professional, and social endeavors coupled with proper concern for their separate needs as well as their interdependence. While there are major flaws within the structure of existing public mental hospitals, until more knowledge is gained about etiology, morbidity, and pathophysiology of the mental illness model, and until societal, cultural-economic, and political attitudes change, community psychiatry—with its emphasis on prevention, rapid treatment, avoidance of hospitalization, social engineering, utilization of drugs, and paramedical personnel to handle the enormous numbers of those seeking help—will not be able to act independently.

In a large measure the programs of treatment and research originating and carried out in public mental hospitals, have contributed to the present state of affairs. Programs of drug research leading to effective control of psychiatric symptoms together with a greater public acceptance of the mentally ill—as witnessed by the open door policy—have permitted an increased rate of discharge of patients into community placement. The resultant decrease in hospital population has led to the naive belief by some that all mental health problems can now be handled without resorting to hospitalization and that if patients are treated actively and early, we can prevent long-term morbidity and avoid the chronicity which psychiatric hospitals encourage.

The role of hospitalization in the United States has significantly changed statistically in the past 15 years. A decreasing rate of inpatients together with an increasing rate of outpatients would indicate that the emphasis is shifting from hospital to community. From a high point of 554,000 patients in 1954 the resident mental hospital population has decreased to approximately 363,000 in 1969. One can only speculate how far this declining trend will continue but one cannot expect it to go on indefinitely. Close examination of the patterns of decrease shows that even now a substantial proportion of admissions are becoming permanent residents of mental hospitals. Recent figures demonstrate that during the past 13 years total admissions to public mental hospitals have almost doubled despite major emphasis on community orientation and a variety of preventive measures. Much of this stems from contemporary sociocultural environmental influences which at the present time are beyond the control of any psychiatric resource.

THE "SOCIAL BREAKDOWN" SYNDROME

Modern emphasis on community psychiatry as a desirable treatment modality received considerable impetus approximately 10 years ago. *Institutional Neurosis* (2), published in 1959, stated that a mental hospital may not only fail to help a patient but may indeed create an additional disorder. Two main points were made. First, this new condition is induced by the institution and superimposed on whatever disorder brought the patient to the hospital; and second, it is treatable and reversible. The American Public Health Association (3) published a volume in 1962 in which a phrase was coined— the "social breakdown" syndrome. This syndrome was said to be exceedingly common in hospitalized mental patients but was responsive to improvement in environmental and organizational services. It has three major patterns: (1) withdrawal of the patient into himself, (2) anger and hostility, and (3) some combination of these two. This was exemplified by the withdrawn patient who was unresponsive to the world and his immediate environment, refused to take part in work, rejected social interactions, was sloppily dressed and disheveled, and demonstrated anger and hostility by being quarrelsome and verbally and physically aggressive. That this exists and could have been effectively dealt with by suitable staff, adequate budget, and public concern cannot be denied. Nevertheless, in the absence of appropriate staffing, with minimal funding and overwhelming numbers of patients, efforts to counteract this phenomenon were to no avail. Proponents of the community mental health concept seized upon this issue to denigrate hospital practice, and asserted that the avoidance of hospitalization would prevent development of this phenomenon. As the community mental health programs grew, there was a rapid awareness of the major shortage of mental health professionals. With the development of clinics—some of them walk-in store front type—short-term treatment facilities, and the expansion of services for emotional disorders associated with social deviance, there was a scramble for services of available personnel, with the result that personnel, formerly in short supply in the public mental hospitals, became even more scarce by their wholesale raiding for service in the community mental health services. Thus, we now face the problem of multiple psychiatric services none of which is adequately staffed. Patients either must wait for longer periods before being treated or, in the case of in-patients, be served by a dwindling number of trained professionals.

What is becoming obvious now is that the social breakdown syndrome is not unique to the mental institution. As the community mental programs develop, there is a growing awareness that this syndrome occurs not only in a hospital environment but also arises from socio-economic factors in deprived and depriving communities. The community mental health facilities deal primarily with low-income populations in which poverty becomes permanent and self-perpetuating, precipitating social disintegration and inhibiting or even preventing effective treatment response. One sees the social breakdown syndrome and other related psychologic states in the community mental health clinic because sociocultural disintegration has been added to the situation.

THE CONTROVERSY

Treatment of the mentally ill has to some extent become polarized. On the one side we have adherents to the concept of public mental hospitals as the basic resource for treatment; on the other, we have groups who feel the public mental hospital is an anachronism and patients should be treated in a community setting with hospitalization almost completely avoided. Each faction can justify their views and quote figures relative to numbers of patients treated, cost per patient, and so forth. Some feel that the public mental hospital should give way to psychiatric facilities in general hospitals. The conflict regarding types of available treatment facilities has resulted in competition for the limited amount of available funds, with arguments presented by all participants being highly biased and demonstrating a lack of understanding of the need for all available services. The public will be sorely hurt if any facilities are discontinued or de-emphasized in favor of the others. The adherents of community psychiatry emphasize keeping patients outside the hospital, close to home, and on the job. This is proper and appropriate for some patients. Those who argue for community based psychiatric services in general hospitals must contend with lack of available beds, competition from medical and surgical staffs, and an orientation which is attuned to the acutely ill rather than to the chronic patient. This situation is suitable for certain types of patients with short-term illness and limited degrees of psychopathology; the public mental hospital serves the chronic patients and those whose symptoms are uncontrollable except under the most stringent conditions.

Additional reasons which are frequently given for avoiding commitment to public mental hospitals are that hospitalization is said (1) to offer the patient a great deal of dependency gratification and remove responsibility from him for his behavior and for the conduct of his existence; (2) to reinforce his experience of failure; (3) to convert him from a struggling, marginally functioning individual to one who accepts chronic patienthood, passivity, and failure; (4) to enhance those manifestations of illness which are caused by alienation from society; (5) to demonstrate to the patient that the therapist does not know what else to do; (6) to remove the patient from reality; (7) to create a social stigma; and (8) to be too expensive (4).

While it is true that there is some validity in each of these reasons, the fact remains that except for the latter two, each can be construed as being a therapeutic rather than an antitherapeutic factor. The pressures and stress of everyday life often require a separation from the provocative environment much in the same way that a cardiac patient requires a period of recuperation before returning to active work.

The primary physician and the community mental health facilties serve as reasonably effective screening devices through which individuals who lose their emotional equilibrium as a result of a variety of stresses (such as a change in work status, physical changes attending illness, breakup of family or loss of a loved one, and economic decompensation) can be treated in circumstances which do not disrupt their daily activities and permit them to remain close to home and family with a minimum of social dislocation. It is when these efforts fail in spite of the active use of drugs, psychotherapy, milieu therapy, and attempts at psychosocial manipulations that a plea for consideration of psychiatric hospitalization is made. If, in spite of the best available outpatient care, the patients' suffering and emotional decompensation increase, removal from his environment may be necessary to bring symptomatic relief. Patients with self-destructive impulses which cannot adequately be controlled in the community may have to be hospitalized as a life-saving procedure. There are others whose destructiveness and aggression seriously endanger the lives of others to the point where hospitalization becomes a necessary precaution.

It is apparent that patients now entering public mental hospitals are sicker in terms of total pathology than those admitted in the past because they were resistant to available care and did not respond to the varying treatment modalities. The current philosophy is that treatment in a mental hospital is a last resort when all outpatient therapeutic resources have been exhausted. Therefore, the major goal for these patients is to create a treatment facility and the environmental support which will shorten the period of decompensation and permit them to return to the community for further care as soon as possible. Unfortunately, the public mental hospital, if it is to be utilized as an emergency device for the psychiatric treatment of a limited number of patients for a short period of time, must have certain characteristics which, in the older public mental health hospitals, do not always exist. For optimum utilization, the hospital should be located where it can be properly staffed; it must be close to a large community from which a full-time staff of competent psychiatrists can be recruited and where the shortage of nurses and attendants, a chronic problem in remotely situated hospitals, can be overcome.

ROLE OF VARIOUS MODALITIES

There is a place for all modalities of treatment. The public mental hospital is a resource which, for the foreseeable future, cannot be replaced or substituted. The community mental health programs must work hand in hand with the public mental hospitals. The techniques developed in these dynamic community mental health programs will serve as catalysts for improving techniques in the public mental hospitals. The community mental health programs will offer the first type of therapy. In time, as adequate numbers of mental health workers become available, effectiveness of therapy within the present limitations will be enhanced, and through the community mental health programs public acceptance of the public mental hospital will become total. For those whose illness requires inpatient care there need be little delay in requesting it, and newer techniques will be utilized to discharge them as rapidly as possible.

The public mental hospital has a unique role in being the only facility able to manage in a potentially adequate manner the problems of severe recurrent and chronic disabling mental diseases. Patients with conditions such as acute and chronic brain syndromes and psychiatric and personality disorders make up 75% of first admissions to public mental hospitals. The observation of these patients for longer periods than might be possible in other facilities allows adequate restructuring of their behavior in a manner which might permit maximum likelihood of functioning in an extramural environment or, failing that, permit them to live lives of reasonable comfort in an atmosphere which is understanding, permissive, and nonpunitive.

The opportunities for research in the public mental hospital are unlimited. Because of the relatively stable environment and the ability for the individuals to be observed carefully, detailed information relative to the disease process can be obtained under circumstances not available anywhere else. The public mental hospital remains the major resource where new programs can be instituted with reliability and control. The management of particularly difficult syndromes in children and in adolescent, geriatric, and psychopathic types of disorders can be considered only in the context of a public mental hospital. One hopes that in the future the public mental hospital will gain more public understanding and acceptance. It is expected, and the trend has already begun, that the public mental hospital will become a more integrated part of the community, fully involved in the medical-surgical model, and closely associated with teaching and academic institutions. It will then assume its correct place in the mental health sequence, neither competing with nor replacing other facilities, nor being replaced by them.

The interdependent sequence of primary physician, public and private facilities, special units, community health programs, and public mental hospitals offers the best opportunity for successful management of the mentally ill in the most expeditious manner.

REFERENCES

1. DEUTSCH, A., *The Mentally Ill in America*, Second edition, Columbia Univ. Press, New York, 1949.
2. BARTON, R., *Institutional Neurosis*, J. Wright, Bristol, 1959.
3. *Mental Disorders: A Guide to Control Methods*, American Public Health Association, New York, 1962.
4. MENDEL, W. M., *Medical World News*, Special issue—Psychiatry, pp. 41-42, 1969.

23

Comprehensive Health

FRANK H. LUTON, M.D.

Professor of Psychiatry Emeritus
Vanderbilt University School of Medicine

"Group medicine is a superior form of service. The best way to make full use of the present technology of medicine is to organize medical groups, teams that will practice in health centers. These must be close to the people in industrial center, residential neighborhood, or farm."

HENRY E. SIGERIST, 1958

The objective stated in the above quotation is indeed timely as well as ambitious. Mental health is a necessary component of such a program if the system expects as its goal the total health of the individual. The quotation from Sigerist also suggests that physicians should collaborate with other physicians and health personnel, and suggests a mechanism by which this service may become a reality. In a sense, the remarks by Sigerist in 1958 anticipated the development of comprehensive mental health centers, multipurpose community centers, regional medical programs, traveling clinics, continuing education programs, and a movement toward a closer relationship between public health and mental health.

My comments will relate especially to the need for greater recognition of the role of departments of mental health, departments of psychiatry, and committees on the continuing education of physicians in this somewhat grandiose program. We have the task of treating all who are sick. The term "health" connotes the preservation of good health and the prevention of illness of all kinds. As a result of the objectives set forth above, medicine has had to shift from its

more-or-less complacent attitude toward meeting the medical needs
of the nation to one of facing up to the reality of many unfulfilled
needs which have come to the attention of the government in its
emphasis on poverty and racial minorities. Program Head Start is
but one example.

The mental health needs of the nation were clearly revealed in the
studies of the Joint Commission on Mental Illness and Health. Its
report (1961) made some startling recommendations which were at
once recognized by the Congress and the President as a pressing
challenge. Prior to this report, a congressional act—the National Mental Health Act—was passed (1946) under the sponsorship of Congressman Priest of Tennessee. This set the stage for the establishment of the National Institute of Mental Health, and provided funds
for the training of professional personnel and for the establishment
of two departments of psychiatry in medical schools which had no
such departments. It also granted aid to states to establish clinics,
treatment facilities, and demonstration projects for the prevention,
diagnosis, and treatment of mental disorders. It is noteworthy that
some of the money appropriated for this Act was given to departments of public health for development of psychiatric services.

It is of interest to review some of the significant sequelae to the
publication of the report of the Joint Commission. The Board of
Trustees of the American Medical Association recognized the importance of this document and, through its Council on Mental Health,
organized its first Congress on Mental Illness and Health in 1962.
The Council also recognized a growing public awareness of the need
for adequate mental health services and posed the following objectives in this first Congress: (1) to assess current activities in mental
health work, (2) to focus on definite problem areas, (3) to seek
solutions for specific problems, and (4) to study additional means
for the prevention and management of mental disorders. In addition
to these goals, an attempt was made to attract and enlist physicians
as leaders in this broad venture of prevention and services. Later,
Gorman, Executive Director of the National Committee Against
Mental Illness, spoke of this "fresh approach to mental illness based
upon a wide range of treatment services in the community designed
to keep as many persons as possible out of mental hospitals."

In 1964, Beaton, at the First Tennessee Congress on Mental Illness
and Health said:

"Every family physician must become engaged in caring for the mentally ill, a task that the American Mental Association has officially proclaimed as the nation's most pressing health problem; the general practitioner must be educated in modern psychiatric theory and techniques. With further training, he is the best person to understand the difficulties of emotionally ill patients and to lead them to their own understanding, to work within the framework of the community in which he lives, to cooperate with necessary nonmedical mental health professionals, and to use the subtleties of the patient-physician relationship in the practical solution of the puzzles of mental illness."

No statement could be more prophetic of the situation that exists today as exemplified by the diminishing populations of the large state hospitals, the increasing number of comprehensive community mental health centers, the development of outpatient services in state hospitals, satellite clinics in the large cities, partial hospital services providing day care and night care, unique programs for the training of physicians in management of the mentally sick at the community level, and the push toward training nonmedical manpower to meet the growing needs for services to the sick in order to supplement the work of the physician.

Then in 1966, came the comprehensive Health Planning Act, followed by a period during which these broad concepts were being developed to include physical, mental, and environmental health, and to cover facilities, services, and manpower.

The Act provided a primary phase of planning and preparing both at the state level and at regional levels to enable health agencies, medical personnel, and consumers of services to work out their own applications of these vast new concepts.

Such health measures as the Medicare and Medicaid programs have dramatically revealed the need for better understanding of mental health programs, especially of state mental hospitals and mental health clinics by the other participating agencies of state government—the Departments of Public Health, of Public Welfare, and of Finance and Administration. Every state Medicaid advisory committee should include a representative from psychiatry. The patients who are eligible for mental health benefits in these programs should also have the assurance that they are receiving the best possible treatment.

Those in the mental health field not actively engaged in the planning have questioned the degree to which mental health is being involved in the overall program. We hear about continuing education of the physician, but where and when does education on mental illness come into the picture? How can the treatment of heart, stroke, and cancer patients be considered without involvement of the psychiatrist or the psychiatrically oriented physician? How can a program for continuing education of the physician in emotional problems of illness be related to the comprehensive program? Are grants available? Are those who are planning these programs adequately informed about the need for this?

Too many psychiatrists are willing to stand on the sidelines and wait, rather than participate during the important phases of planning and preparation. How can a comprehensive health program include mental health without active participation of psychiatrists from the planning phase to the ultimate delivery of service?

24

The Irony of the ICU

HOWARD P. ROME, M.D.

Professor of Psychiatry, Mayo Graduate School of Medicine

It is a truism to observe that health-care service is expanding in all directions at an exponential rate; it is now a 55 billion dollar per year industry. In 1950 it was estimated to be 12.1 billion dollars per year; by the end of 1968 it had risen 380 per cent. The demands for the delivery of this service increased at a rate in excess of comparable increases in other areas of the economy. As gauged by the Consumer Price Index, prices of health service rose almost 67 percent from 1950 to 1965; an annual rate of increase higher than the all-goods and all-services categories. Moreover this increase affects all sectors of the health-care establishment. "Radicalized" is a current in-word; it not only connotes change but also the revolutionary direction and place the change takes. The entire health-care system has been radicalized since the end of World War II. A reflection of this is to be seen in the revolutionary changes in the hospital component of the medical delivery system.

For example, the demand for nursing services has followed the lead of the demand for medical services. In partial but inadequate response to this demand, the traditional duties of the nurse have been parcelled out among a number of more or less restricted occupational tasks. There are the broad general divisions of nursing education, research, and patient service in a similar fashion to the divisions in the field of medicine. In the patient-service area, there are the added occupations of the orderlies, nurses' aides, licensed practical nurses (LPNs), and volunteers. The clerical-administrative functions of the hospital (ward) operations have been delegated in large part to a secretary-clerk. Then, too, there is the educational hierarchy: student nurses in training to be RNs, "diploma" nurses, as well as their instructors, teaching supervisors, and nursing school administrators. In short, as medical education and hospital practice have fissioned and produced specialties and their satellite subspecialties, the nursing profession has also recognized the utility and the need of this division of labor.

The hospital as the physical nodal point of the medical Health-care delivery system matrix has become the center of these specialized medical delivery subsystems. It has also become a focal point for community health care, and increasingly it will incorporate all preventive, curative, and rehabilitative services within its purview.

Apropos of this challenge to traditional function there has been a growing, albeit laggard, development in the architectural structure of hospitals and especially of the units that serve these special functions. Thus, "wings," "pavilions," and "units" have proliferated as appendages to the main body of the hospital, each with its own staff of trained personnel and its own equipment necessary to perform its assigned task. But essentially they have been more or less walled-off compartments—not very original in their concept of design.

Thus emergency rooms, medical wings, surgical pavilions, recovery suites, administrative offices, and psychiatric wards were among the first of the specially designated facilities of the General Hospital. When the utility of physical separation into these gross divisions was demonstrated, there followed progressively smaller subdivisions [e.g., dialysis centers, poison-control units, intensive care units (ICUs)] especially designed to provide more efficiency for the convenience of administration, for the medical staff, and last of all for the critically ill patient.

In parallel the biotechnology used in these units has become more sophisticated. Those architectural and operational changes which have been made for the most part have been made to accommodate the physical equipment and only incidentally the people they accommodate. These costly products have become obligatory equipment for large general hospitals. One observer has editorialized to the effect that the resulting scene is an "encounter not easily forgotten in the science-fiction setting of a coronary ICU. Surrounded by weird electronic equipment, facing anxious fellow patients, nurses, and attending staff, the patient is made constantly aware of the proximity of death" (1).

The designers and indeed the caretakers who work in these ICUs point to the obvious benefits to be derived from the constant vigilance that is available, the provision of skilled nursing care as a consequence of specialization. They are rightfully proud of the lessened morbidity and lowered mortality which follows from the capacity to monitor with the most advanced technologic equipment minute changes in the vital signs and functions of their patients. They consequently avoid otherwise disastrous complications. Then, too, there are other more peripheral benefits such as the economy to the hospital in allocating this expensive equipment to the place where it can get maximum use. In turn, it is said that these economies are passed on to the patient-customer; at least the rate of increase in the cost of hospital care is attenuated. Better and therefore more complete records add to the general store of medical information about the longitudinal course of not only the patient's continuing progress but also critical disease states or injuries in general as well as their complications.

But as Emily Dickinson wryly observed: ". . . We must an anguish pay/in keen and quivering ratio . . ." for every boon. Patients as well as their caretakers who are the subjects as well as the participant-observers of these lifesaving procedures have to endure a certain amount of emotional stress incidental to being exposed to the very environment that will help spare these lives (2)! For instance, Feindel in writing of the selection of nurses for this duty says " (They) should be able to control their emotions. . . . tolerate stress . . . act effectively . . . use good judgment in emergencies. . . ." There have been many studies of untoward psychiatric consequences experienced on the nether side of the bed. Thus, this is a quality of mercy that affects him that gives and him that takes.

The etiology of these untoward psychiatric reactions of patients has been much debated: whether these reactions are in response to some coincidental physiologic insult, or are the consequence of the emotional stress of being exposed to "the science fiction setting." Perhaps it is in response to being subjected to a combination of both ordeals.

The standard procedure that obtains in most ICUs is that regardless of their status as private or ward patients, the patients are assigned to the care of the house and attending staff managing that service which means that whatever their competence technically, this is an entire group of strangers. The ICU cubicle where the patient is bedded is a segment of a larger unit. There is usually a large defibrillator with the array of syringes, needles, and stands holding parenteral solutions. The unit is equipped with a bank of electronic devices for monitoring: tape recorders, an oscilloscope that constantly displays electrocardiographic signals. There may be an additional attachment to permit analogic conversion of heart signals to an audio mode and thus warn the nearby attendants of the sudden development of a cardiac arrhythmia. Inadvertently this also alerts the patient.

The typical ICU patient has an intravenous needle in place and consequently that arm (at least) is tied down. The side rails of the bed are up in place. An oxygen mask with one kind or another of the automatic breathing devices stands nearby. Depending on the size and crowded state of the unit, man and women are in the same room although separated by a curtain said to be "the dirtiest piece of linen in the hospital" (3). Although there are windows surrounding the patient making privacy an impossibility, often the cubicle is kept dark or, in the case of neurosurgical ICU, lighted 24 hours daily. The net result of either of these procedures is that the ambience they create conduces to disorientation. This potential confusion is enhanced by the fact that no radios or televisions are permitted and visitors, one per patient, are permitted for a maximum of five minutes per hour. The anxiety fulminated by these short-lived exposures ricochets from the patient to his family.

There is a flurry of nurses hovering in the immediate area as well as house-staff members within calling distance at all times, since emergencies of a serious nature occur frequently. These obviously require the presence of a team with a resulting increase in the "white" noise level environment and inevitably a subliminal communicated indistinct and unfocused atmosphere of excitement. To the conscious patient living in this environment, the general atmosphere vibrates with an aura of intense alertness. Periodically persons speak (literally) about the patient in muted tones at the foot of his bed but the message that comes through to him with high-fidelity is concern— also present is the specter of sudden death.

As soon as one patient is deemed well enough, he is moved, and another seriously ill patient takes his place. There is an omnipresent background of sound: muffled voices, grunts, stertorous breathing, moaning, retching, and crying. This serves as a backdrop for the periodic interruptions of a troubled sleep by routine nursing chores: temperature taking, the recording of blood pressure, giving of medications, plus the hygienic needs of very sick persons.

While the character of the ICU depends upon the kind of patient it specializes in caring for, the effect upon the nurses is, in the overall, generally the same regardless of their special duties. In order to dilute the emotional impact of this total immersion in critical sickness, depending on their personality, the attendants—particularly the nurses who are assigned to this station on a regular shift basis and who have the most to do with the personal care of these patients— shield themselves from anxiety by delivering their ministrations with a certain degree of emotional detachment. One can speculate as to the probable reasons for this anxiety. Manifestly, constant exposure to impact of death requires a defense. This is a companion reaction to the defense mechanisms used by patients exposed to the same likelihood and circumstances. La Rochefoucauld remarked, "One can no more look steadily at death than at the sun." Hence, the most conservative tactic is avoidance—a resort by which everyone who is exposed similarly escapes from a direct confrontation and thus helps deny the plaguing existential question: To be or not to be?

Although duty in an ICU is similar to, it is also a different psychologic experience than that which surgical teams are exposed to routinely. All patients in an operating room are unconscious. Except for the exposed operative site, the body of the patient is draped. The surgical procedure is never more than hours in duration at most— never days. Although death here too is an ever-present contingency, its actual occurrence is infrequent as compared with the mortality of patients in ICUs. Then, too, upon death in the operating room the surgical team is relieved of the preburial preparations and the family discussion and explanations that are incumbent upon the ICU nurses.

REFERENCES

1. Editorial: *J.A.M.A.*, 205:697-698, 1968.
2. Druss, R. G., & Kornfeld, D. S., *J.A.M.A.*, 201:291-296, 1967.
3. "Building for Tomorrow's Medicine," *Medical World News*, 10:30-35, 1969.

25

National Health Insurance: Will Psychiatry Be Dragged Screaming into the 1970s?

ROBERT W. GIBSON, M.D.

Medical Director, Sheppard and Enoch Pratt Hospital (Balt.)

Within the past decade our nation has asserted that health is a basic human right. But attempts to make health care available to all have been singularly unsuccessful and may even have brought new problems. The most ambitious attempts to fulfill the pledge of health care for everyone—Medicaid and Medicare—basically provided dollars to pay for the services.

This dollars approach was based on the assumption that an adequate health care system existed and all that was needed was money to buy in. Billions of dollars, even more than predicted, were provided but results have been extremely disappointing. Indeed, in many instances we seem to be losing ground. Evidence keeps accumulating that dollars are not enough to do the job; we just do not have the capability to make good the pledge.

This is a terrible blow for a nation that has rightfully taken pride in its medical accomplishments. Our scientific discoveries, technical achievements, and advanced health facilities have been the wonder of the medical world. Graduates of foreign medical schools have clamored for training in this country. Despite these accomplishments there have been many indications that our delivery of health services has lagged. For example, the United States ranks fourteenth in infant mortality, twelfth in maternal mortality, eighteenth in life expectancy of men, and eleventh in life expectancy of women. Certain segments of our population, particularly the black and lower socioeconomic groups, fare even worse.

Several explanations have been offered for the deficiencies in the delivery of health services. Medical personnel is unevenly distributed, notably geographically, but also among specific socioeconomic groups. There has been a lack of planning and coordination within the health care system. Comprehensive health planning is justifiably receiving increasing emphasis because without it there is no hope of solving the health care crisis.

Many believe that health facilities are poorly managed, particularly in comparison with industry. To some extent this may be true, but critics of the health care system usually ignore the special demands that must be met. High quality services even on an emergency basis, continuity of care while allowing the individual freedom of choice, sensitivity to anxieties related to illness, and maintenance of human dignity are all rigorous requirements which add to cost when fulfilled. The assembly line approach of industry in cutting costs would be intolerable in medicine.

National health insurance has been proposed not just as a method of paying hospital and doctors' bills but as a mechanism for change in the delivery system. There are so many complex plans under consideration that it would be futile to speculate as to what form national health insurance will eventually take. Presumably there will be attempts to achieve a redistribution of health personnel, which will include changes in their patterns of practice. Efforts will be made to introduce modern management techniques. There will be an attempt to coordinate the various services by some control mechanism at local, regional, and national levels.

Unquestionably, there will be changes, and major ones. These will be designed with the intent of changing the delivery system to have increased capability of providing care, be more truly comprehensive, readily accessible to all people, and to provide all this at "reasonable" costs. Attempts to regulate other complex systems have been so traumatic, and in some instances disastrous, that we are entitled to view the future with some apprehension.

None of the sponsors of national health insurance plans have been specific about mental health services. Informal discussions indicate that such coverage may be minimal. Exclusion of the patient with a psychiatric illness has been a long tradition in health insurance programs; higher potential costs and emphasis on state responsibility are the reasons usually cited.

A new argument against coverage for psychiatric illness under national health insurance is that psychiatry does already have a system for the delivery of mental health services—the state mental hospitals. Furthermore, an innovative system is being implemented through comprehensive community mental health centers. There is some truth in these assertions but there is also accumulating evidence that the state hospitals, under the impact of rising costs and tightened budgets, are losing ground. The community mental health centers have their own problems, including uncertain financial support at the federal level. No group trying to develop a national health insurance plan should dismiss mental health services on the assumption that the needs are already being met.

If national health insurance excludes coverage for mental health services, we can expect a further breakdown of an already deteriorating system. If the coverage is designed with an overriding emphasis on holding down costs, we may find that little more can be provided than brief, emergency interventions aimed only at symptom relief. It would be far more desirable for national health insurance to make it possible for all persons to receive a full range of psychiatric care appropriate to their needs within realistic limits. As psychiatrists we must take a hard look at the major criticisms leveled against the health care system—poor distribution of manpower, poor management, and lack of comprehensive planning.

Over 40 per cent of psychiatrists' effort is expended in private office practice, with a heavy preponderance in metropolitan areas. By contrast, only about three per cent goes into community mental health programs despite ambitious attempts to develop these centers in the past few years. The private practice of psychiatry with an emphasis on psychotherapy is an approach toward which I have a strong personal commitment, but we must acknowledge that this pattern of practice is not well suited to solving the current crisis. It is difficult for the privately practicing psychiatrist to handle emergencies, to treat patients with relatively severe disturbances, and to reach large numbers.

Most state hospital systems were developed to deliver types of services that are now being de-emphasized. These state systems represent enormous capital investments. In many cases they are hampered by archaic legal and administrative regulations that no longer fit the current practice of psychiatry. The location of the institutions, the organizational planning, and the staffing patterns in many instances are not designed to meet the current situation. At the same time these institutions offer a psychiatric resource with enormous potential which we must make a concerted effort to utilize effectively.

Representing a new approach, the comprehensive community mental health centers offer a remarkable opportunity for comprehensive planning. It is far easier to incorporate newly developing facilities into an evolving plan than it is to change well-established institutions to fit a new and untried blueprint. Nevertheless, we still have difficult questions before us. Should our emphasis be on comprehensive health, as contrasted to mental health, facilities? How are we effectively to engage the consumer in the planning process? How far should psychiatrists go in trying to deal with the problems of society as they relate to mental illness? At what point have we gone so far beyond our sphere of expertise that we have diluted our effort?

These are extremely difficult questions. It is easy to turn away from these issues feeling, with some justification, that our efforts are providing a needed service. There are many ways to become involved on a token basis, such as serving on a committee to write a position paper, being an occasional consultant, serving an hour or two a week in a clinic. However, it is going to take a more vigorous effort requiring real commitment. If psychiatrists are to play a leadership role, they will have to seek ways in which they can actively participate in the various community and preventive approaches to psychiatry. If we don't, others will!

Section IV
NATURE OF PSYCHIATRY

26

What Is a Psychiatrist?

HERBERT C. MODLIN, M.D.

Director, Department of Preventive Psychiatry;
Director, Division of Community Psychiatry
The Menninger Foundation

Recently a psychologically sophisticated internist backed me into a corner with this challenge: "Can you psychiatrists really justify your existence?" He went on to say,

As we improve our teaching in medical schools and nonpsychiatric residencies, most family practitioners, internists, obstetricians, and pediatricians can prescribe tranquilizers, energizers, sedatives, and other psychopharmacologic agents as effectively as psychiatrists—and often with better follow-up, long-range observations and supervision of patients. It has already been demonstrated that psychotherapy is not the private preserve of psychiatry, and that many besides psychiatrists do it very well. Some of the leading lights in your psychoanalytic movement are not M.D.s. In fact, isn't it true that in many instances thorough medical indoctrination may be a handicap in learning the psychotherapist's role? Don't you fellows say that your new residents have some "unlearning" to do before they can do good long-term psychotherapy? As far as community psychiatry and social action are concerned, is the psychodynamically trained psychiatrist really cut out to be the leader? A sufficiently motivated social psychologist or psychiatric social worker can probably do a better job. Why shouldn't I assume that you psychiatrists will be as dead as the dodo bird in another generation? Who needs you?

His questions and remarks were half facetious but, unfortunately, *only* half facetious. At the moment of our impromptu conversation

I was unready to present well-considered refutation to squelch this brashness; I have seriously pondered it since. Concerning our place, importance, and relevance in the social system, my thoughts substantially reflect experiences in my own work. One reflection pertains to efforts involving the presentation of community and social psychiatry concepts to second- and third-year psychiatric residents. Most training programs emphasize psychological approaches to what are conceptualized as essentially psychologic disorders. The traditional treatment modalities taught focus on the psychiatric hospital and the psychotherapeutic interview. The competent psychiatrist-physician uses any method available that might help his patient—from lobotomy to penicillin—whether it neatly fits his pet theoretical model of human deviance or not. At the same time the predominant illness-alleviating measures characteristic of psychiatry are the therapeutic use of a structured environment and the therapeutic use of self.

With the bulk of his training occurring within the medical model and the one-to-one relationship, the resident, struggling for identity as a psychiatrist, leans heavily on the settings and techniques of traditional, established, sanctioned role behavior. Apposing one's self on a hospital ward or in the physician's office to a fellow human being specifically classified as "a patient," best conduces one's clarification of his own role.

The resident reluctantly relinquishes those trappings of professionalism which helped him to the realization of his psychiatric identity. In community psychiatry work considerable modification must occur, not only in the psychiatrist's functions and professional behavior, but also in the settings and techniques required to effect a bettering change. The interested resident is disconcerted upon discovering that effective practice of community psychiatry requires expertise in the therapeutic use of others as well as of self. As Brody pointed out in a Psychiatric Forum (Chapter 31), maintenance of the psychotherapist's model is a serious obstacle to professional community involvement.

In reassuring the residents that community psychiatry is a respectable and legitimate branch of our specialty, I have urged them to evaluate a psychiatrist's professional identity by what he is as much as by what he does. His knowledge and skills should be applicable to a variety of settings and goals. This stance has forced me to define the actually basic knowledge and skills of the psychiatrist apart from any particular social system, model, or role.

In a demonstration clinic in a low-income area we are increasing our corps of nonprofessional neghborhood workers—another experience affecting my thoughts. From observing the interaction between these newcomers and the mental health professionals, we have been trying to determine those functions which only the certified professional is qualified to perform and those which are appropriately transferable to the less highly trained. As our neighborhood workers develop through training and experience, the list of functions and actions strictly limited to the psychiatrist continues to shrink.

From these and other experiences the conclusion is inescapable that professional flexibility is hard to come by. We are bound into a system, a model, and a role. The value of the M.D. degree as currency in the social arena should not be underrated. It's connotations and denotations contribute a number of strengths to the community psychiatrist's position and tasks. Among negotiable coins the following may be counted:

1. A knowledge of biology, normal and abnormal, serving as a sound base, not only for general medical practice, but also for attempts to view man holistically.

2. A special point of view concerning the helper-helpee confrontation, usually designated the doctor-patient relationship. In this socially defined, condoned, and supported dyad, it is assumed that the M.D.-helper is committed to personal service, to a moderate amount of self-sacrifice, to silence concerning his patients' painful secrets, and to a nonjudgmental, scientifically based objectivity toward his patients' human imperfections.

3. The clinical inference process, which equips the physician to assemble, assimilate, sort, select, and integrate a massive quanitity of data concerning a patient into a comprehensible diagnostic formulation and therapeutic regimen. This mysterious process, partly science and partly clinical intuition, is peculiarly important to the successful practice of psychiatry since the nature of our patients' difficulties seldom permits our relying on radiological, biochemical, or pathological laboratories for confirmation and sleuthing aid.

4. Social "clout" in the marketplace contributed to by the beliefs and attitudes enumerated above, and reinforced by legal sanctions, protections, and accountability. Records of Office of Economic Oppor-

tunity programs reveal that often the best and only access to a low-income community is accomplished through offering medical services because the motives for intrusion of the physician and his associates are less suspected and more trusted than those of any other social service personnel.

Leaving aside these medical assets, there is another set of knowledge, skills, and attitudes stemming from his amalgamated professional training which the psychiatrist can bring to the community scene. The following list is not complete nor am I satisfied that it represents my final thinking on the matter; it is a beginning.

1. *Psychodynamics.*—The trained professional, understanding the crucial influence of the irrational in human affairs, listens with a "third ear." He is aware of the importance of separating conscious from unconscious motivational processes, for they must be handled differently. The basic principles of human psychology apply to all interpersonal relationships, albeit many skeptics tend to deny the relevance of psychodynamics as behavioral determinants in persons not labeled "patient." In the professional's view, the recipient of help—be he patient, client, offender, parishioner, job seeker, pupil, or vagrant—functions emotionally and mentally through common psychological coping mechanisms such as regression, resistance, avoidance, denial, projection, metaphor, substitution, displacement, transference, erotization, and self-destructiveness.

2. *Growth and Development.*—The discovery of handicaps or disability is only one of the problems approached by the mental health professional concerned with the several aspects of prevention, correction, and adjustment. The helping task may consist of promoting incomplete growth in many clients rather than trying to change an existing situation. Because of this theoretical and clinical knowledge concerning standard "normal" phases of growth and development in the human organism and the changing interaction of individuals and forces in its environment, he is competent to differentiate arrested development from regression. The professional, in contrast to the layman, having a cultivated sense of the longitudinal life span is alert to the possibilities for awakening and challenging latent growth potentials.

3. *Interpersonal Process.*—The well-trained professional has a sense of timing and process in interpersonal relationships; that is (a) an awareness that a relationship proceeds through sequential phases of

development, and (b) knowledge of how to guide that development —to shift responses and influencing techniques adaptively—as the quality of the relationship changes with changing circumstances over a span of time.

4. *Professional Objectivity.*—The professional comprehends the difference between empathy and sympathy; and his trained capacity to maintain relative uninvolvement of his own emotional vulnerabilities in the disabilities and misfortunes of clients is usually an asset. The professional helper's ultimate purpose is to lead and guide the client to a point of self-sufficiency that makes the helper no longer needed. Ideally, then, the help given has an aducational or maturational component and, at carefully determined times, the delaying or withholding of help is the most constructive move possible.

5. *Interviewing Technique.*—Professional interviewing includes more than friendly conversation, information gathering, or even the establishment of rapport. It involves both diagnostic and therapeutic dimensions. Inexpert interviewing particularly in the initial stages of an assistance relationship, can create serious obstacles to subsequent communication.

6. *Countertransference.*—The mental health professional, through instruction and supervision, has acquired experience with countertransference phenomena and knowledge of how to recognize them; of how to get help, if needed, in using and controlling them. In short, he wears special eyeglasses for looking at both members in an interchange: the professional (himself) as well as the client. He has learned that the source of misunderstanding, misinterpretation, and skewed communication may reside in either or both.

The alert reader will have noticed that the word "psychiatrist" is lacking in the brief explication of these six specifications; rather, they are defined as qualities of the "mental health professional." The psychiatrically experienced clinical psychologist, social worker, and nurse acquire many of these qualities although the properly trained psychiatrist, with his background of medical discipline and psychoanalytically oriented psychology, is the most likely to achieve a full range and depth of all these listed.

The point is that all of these skills can become part of the psychiatrist's armamentarium, to be applied within the medical system or outside it, within the medical model or in several other action models, within the physician's role and the doctor-patient relationship, or within the consultant's role with nonpatients. The awareness of personal professional identity and worth divorced from any single supporting and restricting unitary frame of reference is the surest base for relatively comfortable ventures into community psychiatry.

Have I answered my internist friend's disquieting query? What is your answer?

27

The Seductive Psychotherapist

JUDD MARMOR, M.D.

*Director, Divisions of Psychiatry, Cedars-Sinai Medical Center;
Clinical Professor of Psychiatry, School of Medicine, University
of California at Los Angeles*

A major source of stress in the practice of medicine that is not alluded to in manuals of practice is the inner struggle that the ethical male physician undergoes in defending himself against his biologic urges toward his female patients. Although most physicians can—and usually do—protect themselves against these impulses by having their nurses present during physical examinations of women, countless opportunities for privacy manage to present themselves to doctors whose superegos are corruptible. The physician's conflict is not made easier by the fact that his female patients tend to form strong positive attachments to him, and that the biologic and emotional needs of these women often cause them to take the initiative in seductive maneuvers. The seductive female patient has been dealt with often enough in the psychiatric literature; understandably, however, there has been relative silence about the problem of the seductive physician.

Although no clinical specialty in medicine is immune to such temptation, psychiatrists probably are put to the test more than most other medical specialists because the psychotherapeutic transaction, by its very nature and duration, has a special quality of intimacy and intensity. As I have commented elsewhere (1), the majority of the psychotherapist's patients sooner or later tend to relate to him as though he were a parent figure and to idealize him much as the young child does the parent—regardless of the actual physical or intellectual attributes of the therapist. Such "transference" reactions, moreover, may come from people of considerable achievement themselves. The seductive influence of an abundant flow of transference admiration from such sources may be considerable. At the same time, the usual techniques of psychotherapy, because they generally involve maintenance of privacy about the therapist's personal life and problems, tend to reinforce patients' idealized fantasies about the superior qualities of the therapist. The less patients see him as an ordinary human being, the greater the tendency to assume that he is, indeed, perfect. Patients under such circumstances will often say, "I am sure your relationship with your wife must be wonderful," or "Of course, you probably never have such problems with your children," or "It must be wonderful to know how to handle every kind of situation." Thus there is a tendency to increase the unrealistic aspects of the transference and to foster an unconsciously authoritarian parent-child relationship.

The psychotherapist, too, is often beset by deeply rooted and often unconscious needs that tend to foster or stimulate feelings of physical closeness to his patient. First, there is the obvious factor of the strength of his own biologic impulses. These will vary in urgency at any point in time, depending on a number of elements such as his age, his health, the satisfactory or unsatisfactory state of his sex life and marriage, recency of drive satisfaction, and the relative attractiveness and/or seductiveness of his patient. Second, the therapist's psychologic need to be a helping figure is reinforced by the actual needs and dependency of his help-seeking patient. Thus, just as the patient unconsciously identifies him in the transference with a good and loving father, the therapist's countertransference may stimulate him to respond as a loving and affectionate parent to his deprived child.

An interesting note in the early history of psychoanalysis exemplifies this issue. In the late 1920s Ferenczi, one of Freud's most devoted friends and disciples, began to experiment with more "active" techniques of analysis because of his dissatisfaction with the therapeutic results of the classic method. One of these techniques—based on his ideas about the central importance of infantile traumas and especially parental unkindness in the genesis of neurosis—involved his acting the part of a loving parent, even to the point of showing physical affection, presumably to neutralize the early unhappiness and emotional deprivation of his patients. Ferenczi communicated his technical ideas to Freud, who responded to them in a letter dated December 13, 1931 (2) as follows:

". . . You have not made a secret of the fact that you kiss your patients and let them kiss you; I had also heard that from a patient of my own. Now when you decide to give a full account of your technique and its results you will have to choose between two ways: either you relate this or you conceal it. The latter, as you may well think, is dishonorable. What one does in one's technique one has to defend openly. Besides, both ways soon come together. Even if you don't say so yourself it will soon get known, just as I knew it before you told me.

"Now I am assuredly not one of those who from prudishness or from considerations of bourgeois convention would condemn little erotic gratifications of this kind. And I am also aware that in the time of the Nibelungs a kiss was a harmless greeting granted to every guest. . . . But that does not alter the fact . . . that with us a kiss signifies a certain erotic intimacy. We have hitherto in our technique held to the conclusion that patients are to be refused erotic gratifications. . . .

"Now picture what will be the result of publishing your technique. There is no revolutionary who is not driven out of the field by a still more radical one. A number of independent thinkers in matters of technique will say to themselves: Why stop at a kiss? Certainly one gets further when one adopts 'pawing' as well, which after all doesn't make a baby. And then bolder ones will come along who will go further, to peeping and showing —and soon we shall have accepted in the technique of analysis the whole repertoire of *demiviergerie* and petting parties, resultin an enormous increase of interest in psychoanalysis among both analysts and patients. The new adherent, however, will easily claim too much of this interest for himself; the younger of our colleagues will find it hard to stop at the point they originally intended, and God the Father, Ferenczi, gazing at the lively scene he has created will perhaps say to himself: Maybe after all I should have halted in my technique of motherly affection before the kiss."

Freud's misgivings concerning Ferenczi's technical innovations proved to be prophetic. During the succeeding decades various "more radical" colleagues have indeed extended Ferenczi's ideas step by step to the point at which some psychotherapists have attempted to rationalize various forms of erotic interplay and even intercourse with their female patients on grounds of offering restitutive emotional experiences or of providing a learning experience for naïve or innocent patients. (As might be expected, no figures are available concerning the relative frequency or infrequency of these practices in psychotherapy. My impression, however, is that such behavior is still limited to a very small segment of practicing psychiatrists and clinical psychologists. Nonetheless, because its potential for harm, not only to the patient but also to the practice of psychotherapy, is far-reaching, it should not be ignored.)

I shall not deal in this paper with the various types of eroticized "group therapy" which seem to be increasing in frequency and popularity in recent years, although some of the issues I shall be raising may have relevance to them also. An important difference, however, is that individuals participating in such group interactions for the most part are *consciously* seeking erotic experiences and have some idea of what they are getting into. This is not usually true of the patient seeking psychotherapy.

A significant psychoanalytic figure in these extensions of Ferenczi's ideas was Wilhelm Reich. Although Reich never advocated sexual acting-out with patients, his theoretical views lend themselves, at the very least, to patient-therapist interactions that greatly increase the temptation towards such behavior. Reich's views carry Freud's libido theory to a *reductio ad absurdum*, in which achieving the capacity for satisfactory sexual release, (as the ultimate expression of "genital object libido"), became the prime measure of mental health. The task of handling the transference in psychoanalytic therapy, according to Reich, is that of "concentrating all object libido in a purely genital transference" (3). It should be noted that psychiatrists who were trained by Dr. Reich or by the present training psychiatrist of the Reichian school have been expressly warned against sexual contact between physician and patients (4).

It is interesting to note an American psychiatrist, J. McCartney (1898-1969), made liberal use of Reich's theories to rationalize the most extreme form of sexual acting-out with patients that has ever, to my knowledge, been reported in the psychiatric literature. In a paper published in 1966 (5), McCartney reported that during the last forty years of his practice he conducted "over 1500 psychoanalyses," which means that he "completed" an average of more than 37 a year; yet, according to him, these represented only 26 percent of all the psychiatric patients that he saw! His concept of psychoanalysis may be better understood when it is realized that many of his "analyses" consisted of about 30 hours over an eight-month period, and that their overall average was 89 hours. I need hardly add that, as far as I have been able to ascertain, McCartney belonged to no accredited psychoanalytic society and that his "training" evidently consisted of relatively brief contacts with Jung and with Karpman, a Stekelian, who worked at St. Elizabeth's Hospital in Washington, D.C. for most of his professional life. McCartney reported that of his 825 adult woman "analysands," "30 percent expressed some form of overt transference such as sitting on the analyst's lap, holding his hand, hugging, or kissing him," and that about 10 percent "found it necessary (sic!) to act out extremely, such as mutual undressing, genital manipulation, or coitus." McCartney's rationalization for this form of "therapy" is that "in working through overt transference the analyst should allow himself to be reacted to as though he were a parent. As the analysand progresses through the various stages of psychosexual development, she at first expresses infantile strivings and adolescent needs, but if she is to achieve full heterosexual maturity, she must be able to work through both libidinal and aggressive urges which the analyst must help her to understand and normally express."

The recognition that there is a parent-child element to the transference relationship is indeed correct, but the logic by which McCartney then proceeds to justify an overt sexual relationship between the "parent" and the "child" is little short of remarkable. It is precisely because this kind of unconscious relationship exists between patient and therapist that an erotic exchange between them cannot be ethically or psychotherapeutically justified. Since when is it necessary for a parent to have sexual intercourse with his children in order to enable them to achieve sexual and emotional maturity? Such behavior between a therapist and his patient has all the elements of incest at an unconscious psychodynamic level, and represents an equivalent dereliction of moral responsibility.

Therapists who ignore the transference-countertransference implications of such behavior and attempt to rationalize it on other grounds, such as the importance of establishing "contact" with their patients or of removing patients' sexual inhibitions or fears of "intimacy," simply betray an ignorance of unconscious psychodynamics. Moreover, despite all of the "technical" explanations that these therapists may attach to such erotic exchanges, the fact is that the vast majority of patients invest such intimacies with reality connotations, and hopes and expectations can develop that are doomed to disappointment. As every experienced psychotherapist knows, eroticized fantasies of transference-love often occur in female patients, but when the therapist lends reality to these fantasies by his overt behavior, he fosters serious confusion between reality and fantasy in such patients. The ultimate consequences are inevitably antitherapeutic.

The essential foundation on which the patient-therapist relationship rests is that of basic trust. On the implicit and explicit assumption that this trust will not be betrayed, the patient is encouraged to set aside her customary psychologic defenses and open herself completely to the presumably benign and therapeutic influence of the therapist's professional skill. The ethical psychotherapist cannot and must not exploit the positive transference that develops under such circumstances. Any therapist who insists that this method helps his patients has the burden of proof to demonstrate that they could not have been equally helped in any other way. Otherwise the suspicion will always remain that such therapists are using their techniques to mask and rationalize their own countertransference needs. (It is not my purpose in this brief essay to expound on the variety of inner needs that may be involved in such countertransference behavior. Suffice it to say that it is not all necessarily erotic in nature. Unconscious hostility toward women and reaction-formations against feelings of masculine inadequacy or against unconscious fears of homosexuality are other factors that may be encountered. Obviously, none of these are mutually exclusive.)

Moreover, in the interests of scientific integrity any therapist using such techniques should publicly affirm them so that his patients may be fully aware of this technique before they are caught in the emotional web of a positive transference. To patients who will nevertheless choose such a therapist, one can only say, *"caveat emptor!"* I have yet to see a woman who became involved in an erotic relationship with a therapist who did not end up resenting and feeling betrayed by him. Some of these patients are actually precipitated into psychotic decompensation by such experiences. The counterclaim can be made, of course, that the consulting psychiatrist encounters only those instances that have gone awry. Perhaps so, but the psychodynamics of these situations leave little doubt in my mind that the negative effects must inevitably outweigh any positive ones. Those who argue to the contrary have a professional obligation to publish their "favorable" results and expose them to the consensual validation of their peers.

Still another element involved is the threat that such behavior poses to the professional status of the psychotherapist himself. I still recall the tragic end to the brightly promising career of that gifted psychiatrist, W. Beran Wolfe, who had to flee the country in the 1930s when he was charged with "impairing the morals" of an adolescent girl whom he had under treatment. He was subsequently killed in an automobile accident in Europe with another patient of his.

It is, of course, possible for a therapist genuinely to fall in love with his patient. After all, therapists are human beings and are not immune to such feelings. If and when such an event should take place, however, there is a primary obligation on the part of the therapist to discontinue the therapy immediately and thereafter relate to his patient simply as one human being to another. Any further treatment that she receives should be from another therapist. Having said this, however, I must still affirm my clinical conviction that the therapist to whom this happens has failed in his primary responsibility to the woman who came to him as a patient. I make this statement in full knowledge of the fact that a number of prominent psychiatrists and psychoanalysts have married former patients. I do not know how many others who did not reach this "honorable" end-point have nevertheless rationalized their loss of self-control on the basis of "falling in love" with their patients. My point, however, is that such a rationalization should not obscure the fact that whenever this happens, the psychotherapist has failed to master his countertransference feelings.

Although up to this point this article has been written primarily within the context of the male therapist-female patient relationship, it should not be assumed that sexual acting-out is restricted to this pattern. In their volume on *Human Sexual Inadequacy*, Masters and Johnson report obtaining histories of sexual exchange between patients and therapists from every conceivable level of professional discipline involved in the counselling or treatment of sexually inadequate individuals, including theologians and lawyers as well as physicians and psychologists. Although the most frequently encountered pattern was that of seduction of females by male therapists, they have also recorded histories of male patients seduced by male therapists, of female patients seduced by female therapists, and of "two female therapists who have joined male patients in sexual intercourse" (6).

It is interesting to note that seduction of male patients by female therapists, although not unknown, seems to occur much less frequently than the reverse pattern. There are a number of probable reasons for this. For one thing, women in our culture are conditioned from an early age not to take the initiative sexually, and thus generally are more able than men to control their sexual impulses. Within the same cultural context, women are reared to consider it egosyntonic and virtuous to reject a male's sexual advances, but our sexual double standards provide much less of a protective super-ego barrier to the male faced with a seductive female. Finally, of course, in almost all societies, the incest taboos between mothers and sons are more powerful than those between fathers and daughters. Thus within the parent-child transference of the therapeutic interaction, the barriers toward sexual acting-out between female therapist and male patient tend to be stronger on both sides.

One final question: Can the "laying on of hands" ever be considered a useful therapeutic adjuvant? My answer to this would be a qualified yes—in highly specific clinical situations. In an anaclitic therapeutic approach to seriously ill psychosomatic patients such as those with ulcerative colitis or in status asthmaticus, a "maternal" holding or stroking of hands may be both helpful and justified. Similar behavior may be indicated and useful with regressed psychotic patients. Non-erotic holding or hugging of preadolescent children, especially those who are autistic and withdrawn, may even be essential in their therapy.

With most patients with neurotic and personality disorders, however, in my opinion the psychotherapist should be extremely wary with regard to physical contact if there is the slightest possibility that it might be interpreted or responded to as erotic. Once therapist and patient know each other well and a complete sense of mutual trust and security has been established, a friendly or reassuring pat on the shoulder may be a useful bit of nonverbal communication. But the therapist who does this must be quite sure of his own motives and feelings in so doing. If there is any hidden erotic element in such a gesture, the patient's unconscious will usually pick it up—to the detriment of the therapeutic process. The cardinal rule of all medical therapy applies here as elsewhere—above all else, do not harm your patient. *Primum non nocere!*

REFERENCES

1. MARMOR, J., *Amer. J. Psychiat.*, 110:370-373, 1953.
2. JONES, E., *Life and Work of Sigmund Freud, Vol. 3*, Basic Books, Inc., New York, 1957. Pp. 163-164.
3. REICH, W., *Character Analysis*, Orgone Institute Press, New York, 1945.
4. BAKER, E. F., *Man in the Trap*, The Macmillan Company, New York, 1967.
5. McCARTNEY, J., *J. Sex Research*, 2:227-237, 1966.
6. MASTERS, W. & JOHNSON, V., *Human Sexual Inadequacy*, Little, Brown & Co., Boston, 1970, p. 390.

28

Psychotherapy – Quo Vadis

EDWARD H. KNIGHT, M.D.

Clinical Professor of Psychiatry
Louisiana State University Medical School

It will be difficult for historians of the Twentieth Century to decide which present influence in our culture will have played the greater part in shaping human destiny, the solid impressive advances of physical science or the amazing growth of practical psychotherapy and its nascent progeny, a general psychology of human behavior. The question, as such, may seem superfluous but the possibility of its even being considered today suggests important implications for current problems and opportunities in the field of behavioral science.

Various energetic movements have converged into, and elevated, behavioral science to its present eminence. Among a few are psychoanalysis, its offspring psychodynamic psychiatry, the mental health movement, the developing profession of social casework, group psychotherapy, community and preventive psychiatry, and others. In addition, the study of psychologic phenomena has become increasingly important in such seemingly disparate areas as anthropology, space medicine, industry and religion. Hardly any field in the humanities or the physical and social sciences is unaffected, as the common denominator in all cases is, of course, man himself. In our time, more than ever before, mankind is being forced to come to grips with its main problem—itself. Some contemporary historians even have referred to our epoch as the "age of the psychological (Freudian) man."

Although the pressure to learn more about the mental and social aspects of man, coming from a beleaguered and realistically endangered society, are great and urgent, this need alone would not have been sufficient to account for the burgeoning interest in behavioral science. At the very heart of this evolutionary thrust, both as its major manifestation as well as its most compelling life blood, is the growth and popularity of pragmatic psychotherapy. This simple fact is often overlooked in the rash of clinical and research activities permeating so many of the medical and social sciences. There is hardly a field of endeavor occupied with the study of man that has not been at least touched upon by the "psychotherapy venture." For the first time in history there is available an effective means of deliberately altering the course of an individual's life, frequently with internal psychologic change. As a treatment modality it has been embraced by practitioners of many disciplines, some of whom have hitherto not been particularly occupied with therapeutics. In those social sciences which are not directly concerned with healing, such as anthropology and sociology, its impact as a source of information and a new way of viewing human activity has led to changes in theory, training and practice. Anthropologists of today have employed psychotherapy as a means of furthering their understanding of the psychologic and inner life of their subjects. Many scholastic specialties look to psychotherapeutic data for additional fresh insights, hypotheses and theories that are applicable to their particular field.* Other specialties have been drawn into an essentially clinical redefinition of their professional identity. Caseworkers, clinical psychologists, many clergymen and some educators, have come to view psychotherapy as their major defining activity. Their respective orientations, training and to some extent, styles of practice, may vary, but at a theoretic level the common denominator is still psychodynamic psychotherapy. This had led to problems of professional identity and interdisciplinary bickering.

Inevitably, all students of human behavior have come to recognize that there is no one investigatory source of data from which valid understanding of the complexities of human behavior may be derived. Holistic man is a composite of physical, psychologic, social and spiritual dimensions and cannot be grasped at all if fragmented. Therefore, all applied and academic specialties must contribute to the further development of a general psychology of human behavior.

---

* The obvious impact of psychologic information on the arts, popular and esoteric, is well known and not discussed here.

None may singly claim absolute jurisdiction or professional priority.

This issue is particularly sharp where medical interests are concerned. Psychiatrists feel most entitled to authority in the field of psychologic treatment, by virtue of their traditional role in relation to mental illness and their more thorough training in most areas relevant to psychopathology. By and large medicine (e.g., psychiatry) has the general backing of Western society in this issue, as matters of aberrant behavior are still best viewed via the illness or disease model. Until this perspective or paradigm is replaced by another, it will continue to be the basic orientation of all who labor in the vineyards of psychotherapy, regardless of their particular professional background. There are efforts to conceptualize faulty human adaptation as disorders of learning rather than illness, but this point of view has not taken hold or proven its effectiveness.

Thus, a multifaceted dilemma is posed which may seriously affect the future of the therapist as well as the scholar who looks to psychotherapy for new data and hypotheses. Psychotherapy has radically changed and revised the training, orientation and identity of many specialties, and is the bulwark of psychiatry. In the former case, such professions as social work and psychology have become more medical in their orientation, and in the latter situation, psychiatrists are finding it necessary to equip themselves with sociologic and academic psychologic information. Each of the major groups involved must of necessity seek further enlargement of its perspective through the study of the others', formerly quite distinct, subject matter. The problem of conflicting and overlapping professional identities will never be resolved by simply allowing each of the specialists to continue in separate training facilities; each rationalizing their raison d'être as springing from some historical claim-staking. More important, however, is the probability that the quest for a unified theory of human behavior will suffer unless all of the parties combine their efforts and seek to standardize, revise and legitimatize the identity of the professional psychotherapist. It appears inevitable that, in time, we must accept the field of professional psychotherapy as an established delineated entity and not as a hodgepodge hierarchical jumble of competing subspecialties. All psychotherapists of the future should be comparably trained and exposed to areas of knowledge relevant to the therapeutic venture. Research done via this method of therapeutic intervention must spring from an orientation broadly based and sufficiently integrated so that its findings and results may be useful to all fields rather than labeled or sequestered as psychologic, sociologic, or psychiatric.

This problem may wend its way through the next few decades evolving a solution of its own, or its resolution may be favorably altered or accelerated by planned activity at an educational level. To do this, it is necessary that we thoroughly grasp two current features in the emerging panorama of behavioral science. One is the already mentioned emergence of psychotherapy as a sharply defined and completely new profession. The second feature is that medical science itself is undergoing very drastic changes which are going to lead to the establishment of several varieties of medical practitioners. These two trends are highly significant, organically related, and crucial to progress in the field of human behavior. Each is highly complex and cannot be covered in a discussion of this sort. Nevertheless, an attempt will be made to summarize the important features of each. Enough has been said already about the impact of psychotherapy on various disciplines, including medicine, to indicate that much of the confusion regarding differences in professional identity will ultimately be resolved when psychotherapy settles securely into its position as the applied branch of the pure science of human behavior. When this happens, perhaps some of the social sciences and humanities which have currently been drawn into the plethora of professional clinical involvement may return to their original academic research orientation. Some of the members of these fields may continue their involvement in the applied science psychotherapy as a means of contributing to and participating in ongoing research that is especially relevant to their own particular field. For example, there will be anthropologists or sociologists occupied in clinical psychotherapy for research purposes who must of necessity practice the same brand of treatment technique that is employed in other fields. This will require training, at the applied level, similar to that of practitioners in all disciplines.

Much more complex are the developmental changes in the field of medicine itself. Generally speaking, the enormous information overload and tremendous expansion of knowledge and techniques in all of the areas covered by medicine are making it increasingly apparent that several new varieties of trained medical specialists must emerge. For purposes of discussion, we might suggest that future medical schools will train practitioners in the surgical specialties, in behavioral science, internal or physiologic medical specialists, and specialists in the nuclear-electronic sciences. These four groups are simply suggested to indicate a possible breakdown of the major areas of medicine. All are vital to the continued growth and expansion of medicine, yet the total of findings in all have so overburdened medicine that it is already becoming impossible for a single physician to acquire competence or skill in one area, much less encompass the totality of relevant material.

We may anticipate that the medical students of the future may receive a basic science training curriculum applicable to the four areas of medical specialization. Upon completion of this general medical science orientation, the student would enter one of the major specialty areas, thereafter to receive very little of his further training in company with his preclinical fellows who have chosen other specialty areas. Having completed his period of basic training in the physiologic, anatomic and biochemical sciences, he would then be considered prepared to pursue several years of clinical training in a specialty field such as behavioral science. His previously attained B.S. or B.A. degree would be chronologically comparable to the M.A. of other schools. The remaining three or four years of clinical study and experience, with minimal exposure to other branches of clinical medicine, would complete his requirements for the conventional M.D. Specialized internships could be absorbed into the period of clinical training. Upon entry into a School of Behavioral Science, he would be joined by M.A. students from other disciplines who had determined to seek their Ph.D. specialty training in the area of behavioral science. Both the medical student and the Ph.D. aspirant would continue their training in the medical center, receiving the same courses as far as psychotherapy and behavioral science were concerned. They would each bring with them differences in preclinical training and orientation, but they would share in common doctoral level studies of human behavior and psychotherapy. The problem of deficiencies or differences in training during the undergraduate or preclinical years would require special provision. In the case of the medical student, during his first year in the Behavioral Science Department, he would be required to take certain courses in the humanities and social sciences relevant to his total training, the outcome of which would place him somewhat more on a par with his fellows from the university campus than is currently the case with our psychiatric residents. On the other side, Ph.D. students would find it necessary to take review courses in the physical and physiologic aspects of the biologic sciences in order that they might be similarly equipped to continue their studies in behavioral science and communicate more adequately with their companions who had arrived on the scene from the undergraduate medical curriculum.

We already have something comparable to this abbreviated introduction to the medical point of view in the training that is currently offered to nursing students. It is quite possible that, during a year of intensive review work, students who had received no training in the physical and physiologic sciences would be able to cover material necessary for an understanding of pathology insofar as it is necessary to the psychotherapist. Student nurses are given courses in anatomy, chemistry, etc., which adequately prepare them for their duties on the wards in conjunction with physicians. We must bear in mind that much of their training during the three-year period is occupied with actual clinical services. When we consider that these aspects would not be necessary for the psychotherapist, it is quite likely that a one-year exposure to the chemistry, physiology, anatomy and pathology could adequately prepare the psychotherapist for the amount of understanding he would need to adequately visualize the total patient. Other courses in clinical aspects of illness could follow as the student of behavioral sciences continues his training in the medical center in conjunction with specialists in other fields. The principle involved here is that the psychotherapist must know an essential minimum regarding the bodily aspects of illness and must also be exposed to the vicissitudes of life and death, birth and growth, that can only be obtained by daily contact, training and exposure in the medical environment. In the same sense, the medical student would be better equipped to pursue his studies in behavioral science and psychotherapeutic practice with more adequate grounding in the general principles of sociology, anthropology, psychology and other participating disciplines. We must realistically accept the fact that none of these students could become experts or proficient in those areas which they were simply attempting to sample or review. The lack of in-depth understanding of allied or companion fields of study would be more than offset by the broadening of perspective and increase of communicative possibilities. What is important is that each of the representatives of the various specialties have sufficient exposure to the others' fields of activity so that they might be able to combine and pool their efforts in the latter years of their training in behavior science. One might ask why bother to go through all of this complicated cross-pollination and exchange of curricula when it might be simpler to just continue requiring students of all disciplines to go through the orthodox medical schooling. Such a procedure would inevitably continue the present split among the practitioners and researchers involved in behavioral science.

The student of the social sciences who sought his Ph.D. training and certification in the medical center would also emerge with a degree in medical psychotherapy that would legitimately equip him to practice in the community. If such an individual elected to continue practicing psychotherapy without pursuing further research objectives or providing liaison with his original parent institution or specialty, then at least he would have been better prepared for the treatment of patients. Optimally, however, we would expect that practitioners trained in various disciplines would be in an ideal position to participate in interdisciplinary liaison and contribute special research efforts relevant to their social science orientation. Practically speaking, the medical student would emerge with a degree in medical psychotherapy as well as his M.D. In all likelihood the physician would continue in a role much like that of the psychiatrist, insofar as he would be equipped to handle the somatic and medical aspects of illness. All students receiving the degree in medical psychotherapy would have had similar exposure and training, particularly in the techniques of psychologic treatment. Their background, orientation and perspective to the whole field of human behavior would have been considerably enhanced and unified by the experience of having had their practical training in conjunction with candidates from other areas. Practically speaking, the standardization in the training of psychotherapists would bring much benefit to patients and at the same time clarify many of the professional identity complexities. Equally important, however, would be the results that would accrue from having participants from the many disciplines working together in the medical center in the interest of further research explorations in the areas of human functioning.

It is obvious that innumerable difficulties beset such a plan as sketched here. Hopefully, pointing out a direction for further thought might give stimulus to educators and administrators concerned with the future of behavioral sciences and psychotherapy.

29

The End of "Our" World

PETER A. MARTIN, M.D.

Clinical Professor of Psychiatry
Wayne State University and University of
Michigan Medical Schools

Psychiatrists are familiar with the fantasy met in the early stages of schizophrenia that the world is coming to an end. As far as these patients are concerned, their objective world has broken down, though it is really the ego's projection of an awareness of the breakdown of the inner psychic world. Clinically, one observes that in the wildest psychotic delusions there is a kernel of truth. It was easy in the first half of the twentieth century to see that it was only a kernel and that such fantasies were patently inappropriate to reality. In the second half of this century, the actual presence of this destructive potential makes "psychotic" end-of-the-world fantasies not so obviously out of touch with reality.

Concern about world destruction is a common mass media subject. In such presentations we hear two popular theories of how the world will end. One is the "big bang" theory; the roar of nuclear explosions will herald the end of the world. Such forces may be considered as technological extensions into reality of the destructive impulses of the id. The second theory holds that the world will end with a whimper; predictions of overpopulation leading to famine, pollution, and an uninhabitable environment can be understood as stemming from two sources within the human being. One source might be extreme id impulses toward passivity which resist the obvious call for action to preserve the species. For those who believe in the debatable death instinct theory, such irrational inactivity could be explained in this way. The other source might be passivity or helplessness of the ego in the face of danger signals calling for preservation of the self.

The above preamble is presented to show what this paper is not about and to serve as a backdrop for its focus. It is not about reality, ego and id, and their extensions. The end of "our" world lies in the ego-ideal portion of the superego. "Our group" comprises some young but mostly middle-aged and older psychiatrists. Many are leaders of American psychiatry. Many were in military service in World War II and, because of this experience, returned to the United States after the war for psychiatric training. They carried the attitudes, philosophy, and values of the medical tradition to which they had been exposed and of which they were the dedicated heirs. They were not mere followers but leaders and innovators who, during the formation of the Group for the Advancement of Psychiatry, were labeled "Young Turks." The tradition which they carried even in their rebellion was descended from the classic Greek culture—a tradition of personal development of the individual to the limit of his capacities. Personal standards of excellence were inbred and the individual attempted to live up to the highest principles crystallized within his ego-ideal. Within such principles was Plato's admonition to men who would be wise to "know thyself." To physicians the warning is to heal thyself. The emphasis is on the self, with the concept that if the man is put together in the right way, the world will turn out all right.

It was natural that psychoanalytic training and a personal analysis be included in the training which these men sought. There has been speculation as to why psychoanalysis took such strong root in America (of which Freud held a very low opinion) and not in the so-called sophisticated, cultured countries of Europe. Among the vectors which contributed to this direction in America is the spirit of individualism and the freedom of the individual to direct his own fate. Psychoanalysis meant becoming free, adequate, capable, successful, and wise. The dreams and hopes of the American culture and of psychoanalysis coincided at that point in time.

The group of psychiatrists to which I tm referring was willing to devote years of sacrifice—for themselves and their families—to becoming the most capable psychiatrists possible. Valuing human relationships, they were willing to enter into deeply meaningful relations and to devote themselves to relatively few patients in their medical lifetime. They were eager to become a repository of Western attitudes and wisdom accumulated through the centuries and to treat patients with an approach which stems from the Judeo-Christian ethic: Do not do unto others as you would not have done unto yourself. At this point, American psychiatry was in keeping with the culture around it. Symbolically, the Menninger Clinic—in the center of Kansas, as American as apple pie, imbued with psychoanalytic principles—became a model for American psychiatry. From this stronghold William Menninger continued as a leader of civilian psychiatry as he had been the leader of military psychiatry during the war.

As our nation has changed, so has American psychiatry. The continuing movement from capitalism toward socialism, in the broadest sense of these terms, was reflected in mental health circles. Action for Mental Health and the emergence of community psychiatry followed the national changes. Psychiatry could come aboard and join the movement or be left behind. The mood of the country changed with the advent of weapons of world destruction and involvement in undeclared foreign wars. Scientists previously held in the highest esteem became distrusted. Universities and their faculties became suspect and subject to attack by students. As could have been expected, psychiatry, with its stress on intrapsychic processes, personal growth and development, and sanity is now being considered old-fashioned and irrelevant.

These changes in attitude are being reflected in young residents and medical students. During residency, one can observe not only a relative lack of interest in learning the techniques of intensive psychotherapy and psychoanalytic training, but little consideration is given to undergoing the personal analysis essential to becoming competent in this field. With minimal requirements fulfilled, many residents go into private practice or community psychiatry at incomes or salaries which universities and other training centers cannot meet.

Those psychiatrists most capable of understanding patients' needs through experience with intensive psychotherapy are most capable in crisis intervention, short-term therapy, group therapy, or family therapy in or out of community mental health centers. The therapist is still more important than the technique used. Prematurity, immaturity, and expediency are no substitutes for a solid foundation of training and personal growth and development.

For the same reason, I object to another trend in the training of psychiatrists. Following electives in the senior year, internships for the student psychiatrist will not be rotating but will be limited to psychiatry. Thus, a limited, fine cutting tool will be produced rather than a well-rounded, well-developed individual who is broadly educated in the humanities as well as the sciences. Perhaps this will work for other specialties (though I doubt it) but not for the full development of the psychiatrist.

Future mental health facilities may be manned by mental health workers who are not psychiatrists. Perhaps we are seeing the rise and fall of psychiatry. This concerns me but there is an even greater concern. Is this phenomenon concurrent with the rise and fall of the American culture? Throughout the American scene, are we listening to the death rattle of American civilization?

Is the value—do unto others as you would have done unto yourself —being replaced by an attempt to manipulate others, and, in this process, are we removing ourselves from meaningful relations with patients? Is psychiatry in its responsiveness to the country's changing values succumbing to the growing anti-individualistic climate in our culture? It is clear that the only constant thing is change; but change may be regressive rather than progressive. As values determine a civilization, so declining civilizations manifest a loss of earlier value systems. Sometimes the newer values contribute to the civilization being overrun by barbaric forces whose destructive impulses were hampered by a more humanitarian set of values.

In summary, the group of psychiatrists, referred to as "our group," is observing the end of its world. It is the end of the set of values or ego-ideals with which these psychiatrists were in part inculcated and which to some degree were self-chosen principles. Values have been defined as affectively charged conceptual structures registered by the individual, which act as directives. While a value must satisfy one's inner standards, it must also meet with the approval of the group as a whole, or at least be in harmony with a large subgroup; or one may satisfy one's inner standards even if they no longer meet with the approval of even a small subgroup. "Our group" is faced with the decision of whether to change long-held ideals which no longer coincide with the changing culture, or to maintain them even if the subgroup diminishes. There is little doubt as to where my commitment lies.

30

The Relationship of Psychiatry to Medicine

ROBERT S. GARBER, M.D.

Medical Director, The Carrier Clinic

In the early years of this century, before the rise of the psychodynamic approach to psychiatry, care of the mentally ill was entirely in the hands of the physician and no question was ever raised about psychiatry being part of the field of medicine. With the advent of Freud and his followers and the application of psychodynamic methods of study and treatment, first to the neuroses and later to the psychoses, many physicians and nonphysicians trained in these methods came to question the relevance of medical training and licensure to the treatment of psychiatric illness. Lay analysts treated the same types of patients as medical analysts, used the same methods, and achieved similar results. Clinical psychology developed as a profession originally concerned with psychodiagnosis but, because of a shortage of psychiatrists in World War II, gradually took over psychotherapeutic functions previously considered to be exclusively those of the psychiatrist. Today clinical psychologists are licensed[*] in many states to perform psychotherapy without medical supervision, and their diagnostic and therapeutic techniques may not differ

---

[*] Although medical practice acts in 38 states specify the treatment of psychiatric disorders as part of the practice of medicine, 18 include psychotherapy in the definition of the practice of psychology; 10 have definitions that omit psychotherapy but include "counseling," or "behavior modification"; one has no definition of the practice of psychology but devotes a section to psychotherapy. New York has a regulatory definition that includes psychotherapy. Thus, 17 states offer some legal sanction to psychologists' use of psychotherapeutic techniques. Michigan is the only state prohibiting use of psychotherapy by psychologists, and this is applied only to treatment of the mentally ill.

from those of many psychoanalytically oriented psychiatrists who may use little or none of their medical training in everyday practice; psychodynamic orientation and consideration for the integrity of patients' ego functioning prevent such psychiatrists from performing physical examinations or prescribing medication. Also, much of the psychiatrist's counseling activity may not differ from that of psychologists, psychiatric social workers, or clergy.

What has been described as a cold war has smoldered between psychiatrist and psychologist. The psychologist considers that he has more training in psychologic methods of diagnosis and as much training and empathy in psychotherapy as the psychiatrist, and demands equal rights to practice psychotherapy, rejecting the junior role implied by medical supervision; the psychiatrist points out that medical training is necessary to recognize the organic nature of many symptoms and to use medication and other somatic methods which are often required in the proper treatment of many psychologic ailments. The following abstract (1) is from the American Psychiatric Association's manual on relations with psychologists:

> From the beginning of this report, let it be understood that there are many areas in which little or no conflict exists between the professions of psychiatry and psychology. In a number of areas, there has generally been a spirit of cooperation and harmonious mutual endeavor between the two groups. This report concerns some specific conflicts, and it gives the background for the American Psychiatric Association's official position statements regarding these conflicts in attitude, philosophy, and practice of psychiatry and psychology, particularly clinical psychology, and particularly the area of independent practice of the two professions.
>
> An increasing number of psychologists are setting up independent practice of psychology for the treatment of quite emotionally and mentally disordered individuals and are primarily using the tool of psychotherapy, without consultation with, collaboration with, or supervision by members of the medical profession. (Members of other professions are following suit.) By giving psychologists responsibility in private offices and in public and private hospitals, psychiatrists and physicians have undoubtedly been instrumental in encouraging this attitude in psychologists. However, psychology's growing movement toward the independent, unsupervised practice of psychotherapy has been of increasing concern to many members of the psychiatric profession.

The problem that most concerns psychiatrists is the quality of service to the patient. Ultimately, the person who is suffering and seeking help is the consumer, who should be educated to seek proper help. This should be the guiding principle for both professions, psychology and medicine, in their efforts to change and to relate.

In April 1955, the American Psychiatric Association's Committee on Relations with Psychology published a collection of reports and documents as a reference file for persons who were interested in the history of relations between the two professions. The publication was primarily concerned with legislative actions pertaining to licensing and/or certification of psychologists. Although that issue is still germane, changes in the past twelve years have altered the framework in which relationships between the two groups are viewed. These change factors are varied and reflect growth patterns within both professions, as well as developments of national importance.

The "disease concept" and the "medical model" have been particularly contentious issues and the controversy has been aggravated by psychiatrists, such as Thomas Szasz, who reject mental illness as a myth. The *American Journal of Psychiatry* (2) recently published an exchange of letters in which Szasz enlarges on Dr. Fred M. Sander's views (3) on mental illness and its treatment. Szasz said, "In sum I have tried to develop concepts and methods appropriate to a psychiatry whose problems are not medical diseases but human conflicts, whose criteria of value are not conformity to social norms or 'mental health' but self-determination and responsible liberty, and which is dedicated to diminishing man's coercive control over his fellow man and to increasing his control over himself."

Psychologists have made many important contributions to psychodynamic theory and psychotherapeutic practice; Rappaport, Erickson, and Fromm have greatly enriched the theoretical structure of psychiatry, while in other, nonpsychodynamic fields of psychology the contributions of scholars such as Jean Piaget in child psychology and Heinz Werner in personality development have stimulated a vast amount of research which will prove invaluable in years to come. The growing field of behavior therapy must be considered to have benefited equally from psychiatrists such as Wolpe and psychologists such as Lazarus. At the 1968 annual meeting of the American Psychiatric Association, interesting papers were presented by

Grinker, Sr. (4) and Albee (5). Grinker summarized his presentation as follows:

> I believe that the solution to what has become an endless and sometimes bitter verbal controversy, with threats and lawsuits, is not revolutionary change but rather evolutionary experimentation. All of the mental health disciplines—psychiatrists, psychologists, social workers, and nurses—should be cooperatively involved in the processes of allocated individual as well as overlapping functions. The 1964 position statements of both the American Psychiatric Association and the American Psychological Association include the mutual recognition of competence and genuine collaboration. These words have real meaning and in no way can be defined as depreciatory. The alternative is to follow the plan proposed by Kubie, Mariner, and Charney of developing a new discipline with a special degree under university auspices.
>
> Both models should be studied scientifically. Collaborations between psychology and psychiatry as well as between psychiatry and medicine require study, not explosive disruption. Under any circumstances, standards must be maintained and regulatory devices set up in practice for psychology and psychiatry because practitioners of both professions, isolated from hospitals and clinics in office practice, are hidden from professional scrutiny and are equally open to criticism.

Dr. Albee's paper was summarized as follows:

> This author reviews the evidence for the "sickness" model of mental illness and finds it to be inconclusive. Psychiatry, he argues, in insisting on its prerogatives of primary patient responsibility and control of treatment facilities, bases its justification either on rare and uncertain genetic and metabolic conditions or on the common chronic organic conditions it characteristically neglects; the typical person in psychiatric treatment is suffering from neither. The alternative presented here is a social-developmental model, which would emphasize the nurturance of strength rather than the search for and excision of weakness.

The relationship of psychiatry to medicine has thus in many ways become less clear than it was 50 years ago. It may, perhaps, be clarified by examining the scope of psychiatry as specified by the new nomenclature of the second edition of the American Psychiatric Association's Diagnostic and Statistical Manual of Mental Disorders

(DSM II), and omitting the wider and less well-defined activities of psychiatrists in international affairs, psychobiography, and other areas. A good reference is "A Guide to the American Psychiatric Association's New Diagnostic Nomenclature" (6), wherein the new diagnostic nomenclature, which became official on July 1, 1968, represents a significant advance toward the use of a standard international classification system to facilitate exchange of ideas among psychiatrists of all nations.

Section I of DSM II deals with mental retardation, and the manual specifies causes ranging from infection or intoxication to psychosocial (environmental) deprivation. Most of the causes are well within the medical field, but mental retardation itself has seldom been of great interest to medical or nonmedical psychotherapists; most therapeutic efforts have been undertaken by specialists in education and rehabilitation. This has not been a field of competition between disciplines, perhaps because psychotherapy has been able to provide few beneficial results. This section is of particular interest, however, since it also includes social maladjustment without manifest psychiatric disorder, with subcategories including marital, social, and occupational maladjustment. These are problems in which nonmedical practitioners—marriage counselors, psychiatric case workers, and others—have special competence and experience, although, as their classification in DSM II recognizes, they are often presented to psychiatrists.

Sections II and III deal with organic brain syndromes, psychotic and nonpsychotic. They include senile and presenile dementias, delirium tremens, general paralysis, organic brain syndromes caused by cerebral arteriosclerosis and epilepsy, tumor, and CNS degenerative disease. There is little question that these conditions fall within the field of medicine, and their care is given to the medically trained psychiatrist.

Section III of DSM deals with the functional psychoses: schizophrenia, affective disorders, and paranoid states. Although a few psychiatrists and psychologists may beel that some of these conditions should be treated by psychotherapy alone, most would agree that eclectic methods are necessary; symptomatic benefit is rapidly achieved by medication, electroshock therapy, and sometimes insulin coma therapy. In most patients, psychotherapy is valuable as a supportive measure. Alleviation of mania and frequent prevention of affective recurrences with lithium, without the chemical suppression effects seen with tranquilizers, also support the eclectic approach.

Section IV, the neuroses, has caused most of the cold war between medical and nonmedical psychotherapists. Here the preferred treatment is usually psychotherapy, with behavior therapy playing an important role in the treatment of phobic disorders; the psychiatrist who can prescribe antianxiety or antidepressant medication when required may well have an advantage. Surveys have shown that many medical psychoanalysts prescribe such medications, justifying the theoretical misdemeanor by the practical benefit.

Section V, personality disorders, covers a wide variety of conditions, from paranoid personality and sexual deviations to alcoholism and drug dependence. Many types of treatment have been used with benefit: psychotherapy, behavior therapy—especially aversive conditioning in the sexual deviations—and medical treatment all have their indications.

Section VI, psychophysiologic disorders, requires a physician's expertise for diagnosis of a wide variety of medical disorders, many indicating medication for symptomatic treatment along with psychotherapeutic management.

Section VII, special symptoms, is a heterogeneous group in which management must be eclectic. Sections VIII and IX, transient situational disturbances and behavior disorders of childhood and adolescence, cover areas where psychotherapy may be of great value but where supplementary pharmacologic treatment may often be used.

It must be emphasized that the process of diagnosis by which the various disorders are classified and subclassified in DSM II requires anamnesis, physical and mental examination, and often ancillary laboratory tests, including electroencephalography, brain scanning procedures, clinical pathologic laboratory determinations, and psychologic testing. The latter is not always necessary for clinical diagnosis and is not by itself adequate for proper classification, treatment recommendations, or assessing a prognosis. Similarly, psychiatric treatments include psychopharmacology; other drug treatment for symptomatic relief; electroshock and other somatic treatments; psychotherapy, including behavior therapy and hypnosis; and various environmental manipulations. Two articles entitled "The Cold War Between Psychiatry and Psychology" (7, 8), offer additional insight.

Psychiatrists recognize that the diagnosis and treatment of mental disorders may require the services of other mental health professionals besides physicians. The services of these professionals, when performed in meaningful collaboration with a physician and with the authorization of a physician, should be covered. The professionals who participate in the care of patients must recognize that the physician has ultimate responsibility and legal accountability for the care provided to the patient: the other professionals who contribute to patient care must respect this responsibility and accountability. (Other mental health professionals include, but are not limited to, psychologists, social workers, nurses, and occupational and activity therapists working in a psychiatric setting) (9).

Medicine today is a technology; rather than an art or science in itself, it is a collection of techniques for diagnosis and treatment. The competent psychiatrist must use an eclectic approach with knowledge and experience of many techniques of diagnosis and treatment. Practitioners who confine themselves to psychologic testing and psychotherapy alone are not qualified to take over either the diagnostic or treatment procedures which psychiatry requires. Although there may well be a valid argument for a different psychiatric training curriculum, with earlier and more intensive exposure to psychology, psychiatry at present belongs very definitely to the general field of medicine.

REFERENCES

1. *Committee on Relations with Psychology,* American Psychiatric Association, Washington, D.C., 1955.
2. Szasz, T. S., *Amer. J. Psychiat.,* 125:1432-1435, 1969.
3. Sander, F. M., *Amer. J. Psychiat.,* 125:1429-1431, 1969.
4. Grinker, R. R., Sr., *Amer. J. Psychiat.,* 125:865-869, 1969.
5. Albee, G. W., *Amer. J. Psychiat.,* 125:870-876, 1969.
6. Spitzer, R. L., et al., *Amer. J. Psychiat.,* 124:1619-1629, 1968.
7. Hart, R. H., et al., *Psychiat. Opinion,* 4:17, 1967.
8. Wilensky, H., et al., *Psychiat. Opinion,* 4:30-33, 1967.
9. Barton, W. E. (Ed.), *Guidelines for Psychiatric Services Under Health Insurance Plans,* American Psychiatric Association, Washington, D.C., 1969.

31

Psychiatry's Continuing Identity Crisis: Confusion or Growth?

EUGENE B. BRODY, M.D.

Professor and Chairman, Department of Psychiatry
University of Maryland School of Medicine

What is a psychiatrist?

An institutional answer is not difficult. He is a physician who after prescribed graduate training specializes in the diagnosis and treatment of mental illness.

The illusory clarity vanishes, however, with the question rephrased in terms of role and professional identity. What is the exact nature of the doctor's function? How does it relate to that of other professional people and institutions? How relevant is his educational experience to his role? What, after all, is meant by the "mental illness" or the "mental health" which constitutes his purview?

Illness and health, their definition, occurrence, and consequences are determined in part by social structure. Societies maintain their structures and ensure their survival through mechanisms of socialization and of self-regulation or social control. One institutionalized behavior pattern, part of the social control system of all highly organized societies, is the extrusion of deviant members into jails, hospitals, or other isolation or behavior-modification stations. Even self-motivated consultation with a practitioner is a societally determined response. It reflects the help-seeker's judgment about himself on the basis of learned group standards. Self or other-defined deviants, first labeled as "sick" or "disturbed," eventually become involved in a treatment

---

This question has been examined by the author in earlier publications concerned with specific aspects of the problem (1-5).

or caretaking relationship with a socially designated individual or institution. Thus, they acquire new roles as "clients" or "patients." The patient role, as described by Parsons (6), involves exemption from the performance of certain normal social obligations as well as responsibility for one's own state. Its conflict-resolving value, however, varies in different strata of the social order.

The psychiatrist is part of society's caretaking and behavior-modifying system. Without willing it, he is an agent of social control. He may help broaden or narrow the limits of tolerated behavior. He must deal with the psychiatric fallout, the casualties of the system; but he cannot do this indefinitely without concern for reducing their number. Prevention congruent with his healer's role includes case-finding, early detection, and the rapid initiation of such treatment as he commands. This may bring him into contact with the social system where it hurts—the police, the courts, and the work and living places of the poor. Removed from mental illness, and not part of the psychiatrist's accepted role, though still health-related, are efforts to reduce the cycle of reproductive insult. As emphasized by Pasamanick and Knobloch (7), the elimination of injury and disease in the last trimester of pregnancy, during the birth process itself, and in the first months of the new infant's life, would significantly reduce the warehousing demands on public mental institutions.

Psychiatric roles in the social control system and the socialization process are already well established. Involvement with families, as well as with secondary agents of socialization, such as the schools, is the rule. The area of uncertainty concerns society-wide action which may have primary preventive value. There might be less question about this if psychiatric disorder more clearly fitted the medical concept of disease with precisely identifiable causes; then, the psychiatrist, like the investigators of malaria, could focus his energies on finding the specific agents of illness, and the vectors which transmit them. The question arises when even without this knowledge he goes beyond the role of the investigator and undertakes the job of swamp-clearing. It seems likely that our socioeconomic swamps do contain etiologic and transmissive agents involved in some types of psychiatric malfunction, but it is not proven. Underemployment, powerlessness, lowered self-esteem, and isolation from the information network may be assumed to at least contribute to the probable occurrence of deviant behavior ranging from antisocial acts and self-narcotization to that reflecting impaired reality testing. Certainly socioeconomic factors and their concomitants are primary contributors to such preventable (though not necessary, unique, or sufficient) aspects of the sequence leading to eventual mental hospitalization as reproductive insult, out-of-wedlock marriage, and fatherless families. But does the psychiatrist or do members of an organization which he leads have the competence or the obligation to engage in preventive social swamp-clearing? Should they confine themselves to secondary prevention and treatment? Do they have an obligation to help create a community where there has only been a noncommunity before? Should the psychiatrist, or should the social workers, public health nurses, or other non-physician personnel on his staff become deliberately involved with helping tenants' groups deal with retaliatory eviction, opening channels of communication to the Mayor's office, reducing racial discrimination by employers? Do they have a legitimate and useful role in dealing with any of the stresses which have converted contemporary inner cities into pressure cookers? Is such a role congruent with their functioning as individual healers? Does it lessen the power and effectiveness granted by their traditional socially accepted status? Might it not be more feasible to move the social system through more sensitive employment of their customary clinical and consultant techniques?

These are questions which the safely insulated private hospital staff or the full-time practitioner of office psychotherapy may continue to avoid for a while. They are beginning to approach full boil, however, in institutions, centers, and universities being inexorably pushed toward participation in the neighborhoods and cities which surround them. Thus, a broadening split is occurring in the occupational demands upon and the consequent interests and attitudes of publicly and privately based psychiatrists. The private entrepreneur of psychotherapy, no matter what his professional discipline, has the luxuries of income rising in proportion to the inflationary spiral, of privacy in his office, and of work with people of similar education, class, and subculture. The public mental health professional lives on a relatively fixed salary, is exposed at times to rather traumatic social visibility, and works at the boundaries or interfaces of class, culture, and color. He may deal with the anxiety engendered by this situation through identification with the simultaneously needy and threatening public which his institution is supposed to help. Since his education and background are usually similar to that of other colleagues, and since he himself, especially if he is a psychiatrist, could easily make the decision to return to private practice (in or out of a hospital), his own continuing identity struggle mirrors that of his profession at large.

Perhaps some of the role conflict engendered by these questions might be resolved if the psychiatrist were to revert to the early concept of the physician. Physicians have traditionally gone to homes and neighborhoods; they were known to families, employers, school-teachers, and ministers. In small towns many were community leaders and could move the social system from the top. They have regularly been sought out as sources of wise counsel for problems far removed from the purely physiologic or psychologic. But in the decades since the end of World War II the work of dealing with health and illness has been shared by an increasing number of people from professions other than medicine. This has been especially true for the problems of mental health and illness. Every human being, by virtue of his own life experience, considers himself something of an expert on the behavior of others. Aside from this, the wide proliferation of psychotherapists, counselors (marital, vocational, rehabilitation, pastoral), caseworkers, sensitivity trainers, group dynamics experts, activity therapists, psychodramatists, and, most recently, nude marathon conductors has contributed mightily to the role ambiguity of the psychiatrist. Ambiguity is always intense wherever overlapping areas of function exist, and nowhere is there greater overlap and presumed knowledge than about how people think, feel, and act. Insofar as the developing resident's or the practioner's self-image is that of a psychotherapist (of whatever persuasion), viewed in contrast to rather than as part of the role of physician, he suffers an even more intense blurring of his professional ego-boundaries.

Some of this blurring stems from the organizational influence of psychoanalysis. In no field of medicine aside from psychiatry has a supraordinate system of training, independent of universities and beyond the residency level, exercised this kind of influence. Nor is there another field of medicine in which the practitioner's therapeutic use of himself has required him to undergo a period of patienthood for self-calibration. These features are not, of themselves, undesir-able. Substitution of the identity of psychotherapist (including that of psychoanalyst), however, for that of physician threatens the psy-

chiatrist with loss of the physician's traditional mantle of social
responsibility and authority. Perhaps psychotherapy, in whatever
form, should be regarded less as a profession than as a skill which
may be acquired (including the appropriate characterologic tempering) and used by people from a variety of disciplines.

Another source of role uncertainty lies in the irrelevance for the
psychiatrist of so much learned at arduous cost during his medical
school experience. This, of course, is increasingly true for other
medical specialists as well. It seems probable that modification
of the basic medical training will be accomplished without sacrificing
the professional essence of the physician. This is less his body of
scientific knowledge and lifesaving techniques, as such, than what
he has become through the process of acquiring and using them;
these represent a mode of responsible participation in the social context in which he and his patients live. In passing, it is time to abandon the notion that regularly engaging in physical examinations
or other organic medical procedures is necessary to the continued
maintenance of the psychiatrist's identity as a physician. It is possible, however, that, given the rise of nonmedical psychotherapists,
the psychiatrist's identity problem will be solved by return to the
traditional physician's role. Thus, he would give medicine, offer counsel, and exert administrative authority, leaving concern with behavioral science and systematic psychotherapy to other professions.

These considerations lead to a final source of the role uncertainty:
the failure of current medical school and residency training to offer
the future psychiatrist the kind of education in depth about relevant
aspects of his field available to nonphysicians. This begins with a
selection bias since medical school admission committees favor appli-
cants of proven ability in the physical and biologic sciences over
those with greater talent and interest in the behavioral and social
areas. Within the schools, in spite of rapid changes, traditional cur-
ricular demands are still preponderant. On one hand the student does
not acquire the behavioral science base of the experimental psychologist, sociologist, anthropologist, or neurobiologist. On the other, he
does not learn enough of the techniques of community-relevant knowledge available to the student of clinical psychology or of psychiatric
social work. His skills and knowledge, in spite of the powerful impact of exposure to science, life-threatening trauma, and intensive
psychotherapeutic supervision, do not yet encompass the available,

and leave him at times in an ambiguous status vis-à-vis colleagues in psychiatric social work, clinical psychology, or the behavioral sciences.

All portents point to revision both in the curriculum and the function of psychiatrists. Kubie's suggestion for a doctorate in medical psychology is one alternative (8); if it is followed, psychiatry as a vigorous specialty will probably become extinct and the regressive role resolution suggested above will probably occur. Education for the proposed doctorate in medical psychology includes some of the basic training for medicine, education in the behavioral sciences, and much that is fundamental in psychoanalytic education. It bypasses, however, the legal and related problems to be solved if the graduate is to dispense drugs and assume 24-hour responsibility for hospitalized patients. Without solving the question of responsibility it cannot offer the tempering experience of 24-hour-a-day contact with suffering human beings, as their societally designated helper, which is so integral a part of the physician's development. And in social terms, it poses the risk of loss of the physician's status and, therefore, of his capabilities.

Perhaps the most feasible possibility, now being initiated in a number of centers, is the development of separate tracks or areas of undergraduate medical concentration for those planning careers in psychiatry. This would reduce the required quantity of irrelevant learning, provide basic behavioral science grounding, and allow the prospective psychiatrist once he becomes a resident to substitute other activities for some of the traditional apprenticelike relationship with supervisors. Two years' experience at the University of Maryland's Psychiatric Institute indicates the success of a mixed psychiatric-medical internship, especially for those with prior behavioral science graduate training; this could be an integral part of a sequence, beginning as early as the sophomore year of medical school and continuing through residency.

When a sequence of this kind becomes established it would seem desirable for it to include at least one year away from the routine training of the parent establishment. This year, depending upon the interests and aptitudes of the resident, might be spent in community work, in another university or private setting, in a laboratory, or in a foreign culture. Desirably, each resident should have a period of personal self-scrutiny in the role of psychotherapeutic or psychoanalytic patient. The problem of how to achieve this remains unsolved, however, because of the cost and the relatively small number of available experienced therapists. Whether or not the desired self-scrutiny and personal calibration is achievable through the briefer more convulsive sensitivity group experience remains uncertain. Many who are concerned with the training and characterologic development of psychotherapeutic clinicians and behavioral scientists believe that more effort should be made to explore the specific benefits which may be gained in this area not only from sensitivity groups but also from psychedelic experiences, hypnosis, and a broad range of newly popular individual and group encounters.

This essay suggests a resolution of the psychiatrist's identity crisis through broadening his capacities in the psychosocial field, in a manner congruent with that of the physician's historic role, rather than through constricting his activities to a narrower medical and hospital oriented function. While pointing comfortably to possible changes in education it does not answer the questions concerning the psychiatrist's community responsibility. It only suggests the possibility of responsible community involvement congruent both with his specialized technical function and his social role as a physician. The profession's capacity for self-scrutiny and self-criticism creates discomfort and doubt as to status and function, but such a capacity and willingness to experiment and change are marks of health; and the continuing resolution of identity crises is as fundamental an aspect of the growth of the profession as it is of the growth of individuals.

REFERENCES

1. BRODY, E. B., *Amer. Psychol.*, 11:105-111, 1956.
2. BRODY, E. B., *Maryland Med. J.*, 9:330-334, 1960.
3. BRODY, E. B., "The Development of the Psychiatric Resident as a Therapist, in *The Training of Psychotherapists*, Dellis, N. P., & Stone, H., Eds., Louisiana State University Press, Baton Rouge, 1960, pp. 86-89.
4. BRODY, E. B., *J. Nerv. Ment. Dis.*, 136:58-67, 1963.
5. BRODY, E. B., *Amer. J. Psychiat.*, 122:81-87, 1965.
6. PARSONS, T., *Amer. J. Orthopsychiat.*, 21:452-460, 1951.
7. PASAMANICK, B., & KNOBLOCH, H., *Merrill-Palmer Quarterly*, 12:7-27, 1969.
8. KUBIE, L. S., *Texas Rep. Biol. Med.*, 12:692-737, 1954.

32

Forced Publication:
The Abuse of Talent

RAYMOND W. WAGGONER, M.D., Sc.D.

Professor, Department of Psychiatry,
University of Michigan Medical School.

Good medicine is based on three significant factors, all interrelated and all vitally important. Research and the reporting of it is necessary for the development of new understanding and new techniques. Teaching is necessary if we are going to continue to have qualified participants in the medical field, but neither of these can survive unless adequately related to the *third* factor, clinical service. It so happens that some physicians are not gifted with talent in all these three areas. Some physicians who are very capable clinicians have little interest in or qualifications for research, or perhaps have a comparable lack of interest in teaching. On the other hand, many clinicians can transmit their medical information and clinical know-how to younger associates in unique and personal ways, but are at a loss to transfer this skill to paper. There are those whose primary skill is in various aspects of research, and they, too, may or may not have the ability to describe their work in a clear and understandable fashion.

The emphasis on publication as one of the most important, if not the most important, criterion for appointment or promotion in medical faculties is not only threatening to many young and capable teachers and clinicians but is also an important factor in the publication of much poorly conceived and second-rate material, which is constantly appearing in the literature.

A good physician is well trained to care for patients. His rewards consist of the material and moral compensations that he receives when it is recognized that he is skillful in exercising and teaching patient care. For medical faculties to require evidence of ability to describe these skills in order to obtain recognition in the university setting suggests implicitly that clinical and teaching excellence are not in and of themselves sufficiently important to warrant promotion, but rather that publication is the really important skill.

This unfortunate policy has come to be so well recognized that the cliché "publish or perish" is used with a frequency far beyond its literary merit. It means, briefly, that if you don't write papers, good, bad, or indifferent, then you don't get important academic appointments. When a young physician is recommended for appointment or promotion, the first question to be asked is not likely to be, "Is he a good teacher or clinician?" but rather, "How many papers has he published?" Possibly whichever committee is charged with the responsibility for recommending his appointment or promotion is not qualified to determine the value of his publications. Some committee members may read the material out of a sense of duty, but unless they happen to work in the same specialty field, they are not likely to be able to judge anything more than the quality of the writing style.

For example, appropriately conceived psychiatric material, even when properly described and presented, may be considered as bizarre by a colleague who is used to the more concrete approach used in reporting in other fields of medicine. The colleague may refuse to consider results that can be duplicated only with extreme difficulty. How can one be sure of or establish controls in a study of psychotherapy of depression? Basic scientists describe psychiatry as unscientific for this reason.

The neophyte in psychiatry is particularly vulnerable. It seems to take longer for the young person in this field to crystalize his theoretic position and thus he may hesitate to put his ideas in writing. On the other hand, he may manifest a degree of reaction formation with the tendency to follow some fad in an almost religious fashion. The demand for publication may stimulate this trend with disastrous results, involving publication of essentially useless material. There are very few Freuds in the world, but there are many interpreters of Freud's writings. Some of these have not even read much of his material. Fewer still have understood him. The pressure to publish may stimulate premature attempts to interpret or write on subjects only partially digested.

The results of this forced publication can be devastating. Clinicians who have little or no investment in research very quickly comprehend that they should take their skills elsewhere. When highly qualified clinicians and teachers move away from university communities, patient care inevitably deteriorates. When a young clinician, deeply involved in patient care, is told by an associate that he may have to pay less attention to his patients in order to publish, it simply means that the person making such a statement has never committed himself to the real responsibility for patient care. It is doubtful, indeed, if this is the kind of person who should be teaching medical students, for after all, medical students are our future clinicians and they tend to use their instructors as models.

In general, much of the pressure for publication seems to come from those members of the faculty who have little or no responsibility for patient care. As a direct consequence of pressure for publication, there has been an amazing increase in the number of scientific journals, and the editors of quality journals have such a backlog of articles waiting for publication that a really good article may often wait as long as two years before it can be published. By this time, it may have lost some of its pertinence.

The criterion of publication in evaluating a physician is often expedient, since it is, or may be, difficult to determine his clinical qualifications. On the other hand, his ability to teach can be relatively easily measured in most instances by the enthusiasm of his students, although here again one may find that what is being taught may make an impression which leads to student enthusiasm, but which is not good clinical medicine. It is unfortunate that the medical school administration often finds it difficult to accept the evaluation given of the man by his chairman, colleagues, and students, who collectively should be in the best position to determine the candidate's merit.

The arguments should not in any sense be considered as a diatribe against publication. Certainly if a physician has something worthwhile to say, either about a patient with an unusual problem or a unique solution of a problem, or certainly in presenting a valuable analysis of data or in establishing a new theoretic position, it is strongly urged that such information be made available through publication. The quarrel is with medical school administrations which, in this author's opinion, unwisely use the criterion of publication as the measure by which appointment or promotion is determined.